SO-CWT-287

KETO DIET FOR WOMEN OVER 60

A Complete Guide To Learn What Happens After You
Turn 60 and Why You Should Live The Keto Lifestyle,
with Quick and Tasty Low~Carb Recipes to Lose Weight
and Boost Your Immune System

30~Day Special Meal Plan Included

By

MELINDA FRANCIS

© Copyright 2023 by MELINDA FRANCIS All rights reserved.

This document is geared towards providing exact and reliable information in regards to the topic and issue covered. The publication is sold with the idea that the publisher is not required to render accounting, officially permitted, or otherwise, qualified services. If advice is necessary, legal or professional, a practiced individual in the profession should be ordered.

- From a Declaration of Principles, which was accepted and approved equally by a Committee of the American Bar Association and a Committee of Publishers and Associations.

In no way is it legal to reproduce, duplicate, or transmit any part of this document in either electronic means or in printed format. Recording of this publication is strictly prohibited, and any storage of this document is not allowed unless with written permission from the publisher. All rights reserved.

The information provided herein is stated to be truthful and consistent, in that any liability, in terms of inattention or otherwise, by any usage or abuse of any policies, processes, or directions contained within is the solitary and utter responsibility of the recipient reader. Under no circumstances will any legal responsibility or blame be held against the publisher for any reparation, damages, or monetary loss due to the information herein, either directly or indirectly.

Respective authors own all copyrights not held by the publisher.

The information herein is offered for informational purposes solely and is universal as so. The presentation of the information is without contract or any type of guarantee assurance.

The trademarks that are used are without any consent, and the publication of the trademark is without permission or backing by the trademark owner. All trademarks and brands within this book are for clarifying purposes only and are owned by the owners themselves, not affiliated with this document.

Table of Contents

INTRODUCTION

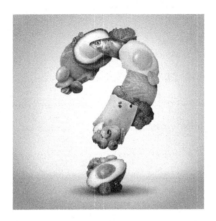

What is the Keto Diet?

Before we get started, it is essential to clarify the keto diet. You've heard a lot about it, and perhaps you still don't fully understand what it is.

Here is a succinct and straightforward explanation of what the keto diet entails.

The ketogenic diet is a high-fat, low-carb diet with amazing health advantages, such as:

- weight loss
- help prevent Alzheimer's disease
- reduce the risk of heart disease/heart attack
- blood sugar control
- helps reduce high blood pressure

and so much more!

The Atkins diet and this one are both low in carbohydrates. However, with the Atkins diet, you progressively increase your carbohydrate consumption. The keto diet, commonly referred to as the ketogenic diet, calls for significant adjustments to your regular eating routine. This low-protein, high-fat diet severely limits all sources of carbs, including grains, bread, cereal, and many vegetables and fruits.

While the keto diet may be difficult to follow, some people find that they experience benefits that exceed their disadvantages when they do. People over 60 may succeed on the keto diet because it may help with weight reduction, blood sugar regulation, and perhaps even heart disease prevention. However, there are risks associated with this diet. Therefore, you should always see your doctor or a qualified nutritionist before beginning any new diet.

What is the Principle Behind the Ketogenic Diet?

We already know it's a low-carb diet with high fat, but what is the underlying science or principle? By starving the body of carbohydrates, you make it burn fat instead of sugar, which causes weight reduction. But keto is more complicated than that. Its main purpose is to help people lose weight, but what about all the other health advantages? Women over 60 need to worry about it because it lowers the chance of heart attacks, may lower blood pressure and can help prevent Alzheimer's.

It's never late to start getting healthy, and the keto diet for women over 60 is an excellent place to start.

How Does the Keto Diet Work?

Usually, after consuming carbohydrates, your blood sugar rises, supplying the body's cells with energy. However, if you go without carbs for a long time, your blood sugar drops, and the liver starts using body fat stored as fuel. It's like a back-up system for your body. We refer to this process as ketosis. While on the keto diet, your body still has access to other energy sources, allowing you to keep your lean muscle mass.

Is Keto Healthy For Older Women?

In my experience, older women face various health issues or ailments. It's crucial to understand that what works for one lady over 60 may not work for another. When it comes to your health, please avoid comparing yourself to others. Keto is good for older women, but you should know that it's also not a very simple diet to maintain. It takes a ton of discipline and willpower, which I don't think I have much. We have been eating a certain way as older adults for our whole lives; thus, it will take a lot of work to alter that drastically, but it will be worthwhile.

CHAPTER 1

Ketosis 101

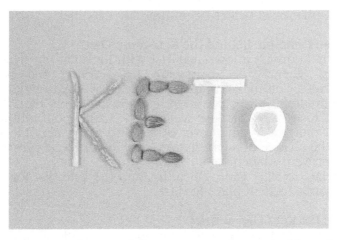

The Ketogenic Diet is one of the most popular and oldest diet plans out there. Although it has been referred to by many other names over the years, including banting, Atkins, Protein Power, and low carb, the concept is the same: limit your intake of carbs and sugars while consuming a reasonable quantity of protein and a lot of fat.

If you are trying to lose weight or just be healthy, you've already looked into this diet, but there is a ton of conflicting information available, ranging from "OMG...this is the best thing ever!" to "eating all that fat will kill you". The keto diet consists of a low-carb, moderate-protein, and high-fat diet. This low-carb, high-fat (LCHF) diet encourages your body to use fat as its main energy source, which leads to weight reduction and a more constant energy level without the sharp highs and lows of a diet high in sugar.

Keto Diet For Weight Loss

Your body adjusts to the keto diet and starts using ketones from fat (instead of glucose from carbohydrates) as its main fuel source within 3 days to 1 week. Ketosis is the name for this metabolic process. When you reach ketosis, you use your body's stored fat and the fat in your food as fuel. Eating delicious fatty foods while losing weight thanks to your body's adaptation to become a "fat-burning furnace" is one of the key attractions of the keto diet.

Types of Ketogenic Diets

While there are many similarities across the many ketogenic diets that have grown in popularity recently, some significant variances should be acknowledged.

Standard Ketogenic Diet (SKD): The most well-known type of the keto diet, the Standard Ketogenic Diet (SKD), is exactly what we have just explained. It is the version that most people follow. When following a standard ketogenic diet, you typically get 70% of your calories from fat, 25% from protein, and 5% from carbs.

Cyclical Ketogenic Diet (CKD): The cyclical Ketogenic Diet (CKD) is popular among bodybuilders who want to achieve exceptionally low body fat levels for shows and competitions.
A "carb loading" day is incorporated into the cyclical ketogenic diet (often once per week) to restore muscle glycogen and boost energy.

The Targeted Ketogenic Diet (TKD): Athletes who need more energy to go through strenuous workouts are drawn to the targeted ketogenic diet (TKD), which is more like the SKD. With the TKD, the person plans their carbohydrate intake to correspond with their workouts to satisfy their energy demands. You must slightly increase your protein consumption if you follow the High Protein Ketogenic Diet. In this variation, fat calories should make up 60-70%, while protein should account for 30-35% of calories. Carb calories are further reduced to under 5%. The High Protein Ketogenic Diet has you "carb loading" with more protein than carb-heavy meals since excess protein takes turns to glucose.

Is The Keto Diet Safe?

If you've looked up the keto diet on the Internet, you've run into a few articles that say it's harmful or risky.
They exclaim, "Eating too much fat can clog your arteries!"
"You won't get enough nutrients!"
All that protein will destroy your kidneys!
You must consume grains and sugars!"
"Being in ketosis too long can be fatal!"

The Framingham Study and the Seven Country Study are mostly to blame for the notion that consuming fats is unhealthy. The Framingham Study is a multigenerational study of residents of Framingham, Massachusetts, which started in 1948 and is still running today. Dr Ancel Keys, an American physiologist who had conducted numerous other studies on how diet affected overall health, was the driving force behind the Seven Country Study, which took place between 1952 and 1957.

This study focused on seven non-North American countries to examine the prevalence of heart disease in these populations. Both studies found that people who consumed more animal fat had a greater incidence of heart disease, but they disregarded other risk factors, including smoking and alcohol consumption. Although eating a lot of fat has been linked to heart disease, this link has not yet been conclusively established. While certain fats are seen to be healthier than others, the demonization of fat has significantly decreased over the past several years. Another bone of contention is the ketogenic diet's alleged deficiency in nutrients. Many people assert that cutting out grains, starches, most fruits, and non-green vegetables would result in malnutrition and believe that those following a ketogenic diet only consume steak, bacon, and cheese.

However, many people who follow the ketogenic diet discover eating more veggies than previously. Moreover, consuming more meat results in more complete proteins and vital amino acids and nutrients like vitamin B12, zinc, and potassium. While it is true that eating too much protein might affect renal function, this only occurs when the kidneys are already damaged. As we noted before, extra protein converts to glucose, the fuel the body use first, which is why the standard ketogenic diet promotes larger ingestion of fat rather than protein. Going keto won't harm your kidneys if they are functioning normally.

Benefits of Going Ketogenic
While weight loss is the main benefit of the ketogenic diet, there are many additional advantages to adopting this eating routine.

Reduced Hunger + Increased Energy: You'll notice that your hunger is significantly less because you're consuming mostly fat and a small amount of protein, both of which are inherently satiating. This is because fat is a more stable and consistent energy source. Furthermore, you'll experience longer-lasting fullness and satisfaction following a ketogenic diet since fat is far more satiating than rapidly metabolizing carbs.

Improved Mental Clarity: Carbohydrates burn fast by nature, which causes sharp spikes in blood sugar levels. These spikes eventually culminate in a crash, which frequently leaves you feeling mentally foggy. Soon, all you want to do is return to baseline, so you reach for a coffee, an energy drink, or a candy bar. Once you start using ketones as fuel, you will soon notice an improvement in brain function, clarity, focus, attention, and problem-solving skills.

Accelerated Weight Loss: Chances are, this is why you are reading this book, right? By switching from glucose to ketones as your body's primary fuel source, you'll soon start burning body fat for energy, which will cause rapid and consistent weight reduction. This is not only a question of speculation or opinion. Scientific research has repeatedly shown that a low-carb ketogenic diet produces noticeably better outcomes than the conventional low-fat diet widely adopted decades ago.

Control Blood Sugar: Since you are cutting out high-carbohydrate and high-sugar foods (which convert to sugar in the bloodstream), many people notice lower blood sugar levels on a keto diet.
The ketogenic diet has been proven to restore blood sugar patterns in people with diabetes as one is essentially avoiding the foods that cause blood sugar imbalances. Many doctors advise Type 2 diabetics to follow a low-carbohydrate keto diet to restore normal blood sugar functioning.

Higher Good Cholesterol: People are concerned with starting a ketogenic diet because they believe consuming more fat would negatively impact their cholesterol levels. Contrary to popular belief, low-carb ketogenic diets have been shown to boost HDL cholesterol while decreasing LDL cholesterol and triglyceride levels.

Reduced Risk of Many Types of Cancer: Cancer affects almost every household in the United States and throughout the world. Cutting processed foods and carbs, when combined with other forms of treatment, has been demonstrated to improve survival chances for some types of cancers.

Digestive Support: For people who experience persistent digestive problems, eliminating or drastically limiting carbohydrates can make a big impact. Many grains, starches, and sugars have been linked to GERD, constipation, and bloating in many individuals. Additionally, it has been suggested that fat nourishes good gut bacteria, improving digestion and stomach health.

Improve Cardiovascular Health: A high-fat ketogenic diet has been shown in studies to promote cardiovascular health, which may go against popular knowledge. This contradicts the "heart-healthy grains" claim that the American food lobby has propagated for years. Studies have begun to show that those who follow a low-carb diet (as opposed to a low-fat diet) have lower cholesterol and triglyceride levels and better cardiovascular health overall.

What Is Ketosis

Your body needs food to function, but different foods fuel your body differently. For many of us, a fast food breakfast sandwich, pastry, and sweetened coffee constitute a typical breakfast. This meal contains a lot of sugars and carbs, which turn into the simplest sugar, glucose, when digested. Before using any other fuel, your body will utilize glucose to power itself. You'll experience a spike in energy as a result of consuming this type of meal. Insulin is a hormone that transports glucose throughout the body for optimal energy. However, glucose burns quickly and hot, which is why you will feel "the crash" and the urge for another cup of coffee, candy bar, or pastry a few hours after eating.

When your body cannot obtain glucose, it produces ketones, a fuel made from fat, and feeds on them. Ketosis is the state in which your ketone levels are raised; once you enter ketosis, you'll experience the benefits described above.

How to Reach Ketosis

Limiting your intake of carbs while increasing your intake of protein and fat is the simplest approach to raising your ketone levels. A ketogenic diet should ideally contain 60 to 80% fat, 20 to 30% protein, and just 5 to 10% carbohydrates. In comparison, the typical American diet recommends 300 grams of carbohydrates each day. A ketogenic meal plan would often have significantly fewer carbs than that, typically between 20 and 50 per day. A diet with less than 100 grams of carbohydrates per day is considered low carb.

Testing for Ketosis

There are various ways to check your ketone levels. The ease of use of ketone test strips contributes to their popularity. One is simply swiped through your urine stream while you wait a little while. The strip's tip will eventually change color. The darker pink the strip becomes the higher your ketone levels. For more accurate measurements, consider a blood glucose and ketone monitoring device, that is more accurate. This device collects blood from a tiny finger prick and provides the most precise blood ketone levels possible. Finally, we have breath ketone-level analyzers. When you are in ketosis, you probably notice a metallic taste in your mouth since ketones are released in your breath. You will likely, at the very least, detect "keto breath," the unpleasant breath that ketosis is known to cause. This is caused by Ketones, which can be detected with a ketone breath meter. While there are other options, we haven't discovered one we love and highly suggest, so we stick with ketone test strips or ketone blood monitors.

Of course, none of this is necessary to succeed on the keto diet, but it may be incredibly rewarding to observe physical indicators that you are in ketosis.

<u>Tips for Reaching Ketosis</u>
We'll go through a few things you can do to hasten the process by which your body enters ketosis.

Eat a Lot of Healthy Fat: You should restrict your carbohydrate intake and ensure you eat a lot of healthy fat. Remember, you should get most of your calories from fat. You'll also be less likely to go for a carb-heavy snack if you fill up on fat.

Keep Your Protein Intake Relatively Low: Remember that too much protein will be converted into glucose, the same thing that happens when you consume carbs. Try to limit the percentage of calories from protein to no more than 25% unless you're on a high-protein ketogenic diet. This implies that you can't eat a lot of steaks every meal.

Add Some Light Exercise: Studies have shown that exercise helps speed up the production of ketones. Indeed, increasing your activity level can aid in putting your body into a state of ketosis. We're not talking about strenuous, all-out exercise, just a little more movement. Walking is a good exercise almost everyone can do, or you can play your preferred sport.

Increasing Water Intake: Water is the ideal drink; while following the ketogenic diet, you should drink a lot of water. In addition to keeping you hydrated, water helps you feel fuller longer, which reduces your need for carbohydrates. Water has also been shown to hasten the removal of fat and ketones from your body.

Try Intermittent Fasting: Since a ketogenic diet reduces appetite, many people adopt a practice known as intermittent fasting. This entails limiting your eating window or missing a meal. For instance, you can just have lunch and dinner and forgo breakfast. While many believe it improves the efficiency of low-carb eating, it is not necessary.

Ketosis Vs. Ketoacidosis

If you have diabetes, you are undoubtedly well aware of the dangers of letting your blood sugar rise too high, resulting in diabetic ketoacidosis, or DKA. If neglected, this severe condition can become fatal. However, many individuals (including those with and without diabetes) may not be aware that a biological state called ketosis is similar and has nothing to do with dangerously high blood sugar levels and generally feeling awful. In-depth explanations of ketoacidosis, ketosis and the distinctions between the two states are provided in this chapter.

What is ketoacidosis?
DKA, also known as diabetic ketoacidosis, is a significant short-term complication of diabetes that occurs when the blood turns acidic from too many ketones in the body in response to abnormally high blood sugar levels. When no insulin is present in the bloodstream, the body cannot metabolize any glucose consumed, resulting in ketoacidosis.

This causes a fast decline and needs urgent emergency medical care. Ketoacidosis can develop slowly over several days due to chronic illness and persistently high blood sugar levels or more quickly from a complete absence of insulin (caused by forgetting to take an injection before a meal or an insulin pump failure). People with type 1 diabetes experience ketoacidosis more frequently than those with type 2 diabetes. In fact, when type 1 diabetes is diagnosed, roughly 25% of people are in DKA. Even though it's uncommon, some persons without diabetes can develop ketoacidosis. Starvation, an overactive thyroid, or chronic alcoholism can cause it.

What are the symptoms of ketoacidosis?
The following are some typical signs and symptoms of ketoacidosis. If you suspect you have ketoacidosis, please get emergency medical help right away.

- Extreme thirst and dry mouth
- Bodyache and headache
- Ketones in the urine
- Frequent urination
- High blood sugar
- Nausea
- Fruity-smelling breath
- Vomiting

- Weight loss (rapid and dangerous)
- Flushed face
- Blurry vision
- Extreme fatigue
- Confusion

How dangerous is ketoacidosis?
Ketoacidosis must be treated right away by a medical practitioner due to its significant risk. If you believe you are in DKA and/or have moderate to high levels of ketones for several hours and cannot lower your blood sugar, call 911 or go to the nearest emergency department. Ketoacidosis can cause a diabetic coma and perhaps death if left untreated. Every diabetic patient should have access to at-home ketone strips to check for ketones in their body (through blood or urine) and help prevent the onset of DKA.

What is ketosis?
On the other hand, nutritional ketosis is a physiologic state that happens when the body starts to use fat as fuel instead of glucose.
The body can use the ketones generated when this fat is burned to produce energy. Rapid and sustained weight reduction can result from this (just like the weight loss seen at the diagnosis of diabetes, but this weight loss is harmless). This often happens when a person consumes a diet with minimal carbohydrates, such as the ketogenic diet, intermittent fasting, or (rarely) the Paleo diet. Nutritional ketosis can be reached after consuming 50 or fewer carbs per day for around 3–4 days.

Symptoms of ketosis
There are several signs that you could be suffering from the "keto flu" or the early withdrawal symptoms from sugar and carbohydrates, even though the only way to be sure if the body is in ketosis is to perform a ketone test.
These include, but are not limited to:
- Irritability
- Headache
- Brain fog
- Cramping
- Insomnia
- Constipation (and sometimes diarrhea)
- Elevated heart rate
- Dehydration

- Sugar cravings
- Muscle aches
- Nausea
- Bad breath (known as "ketosis" breath)

Drinking lots of water can help alleviate most ketosis symptoms entirely after a few days. Kidney stones are more common, a serious adverse effect that some people experience from long-term ketosis. A potassium citrate pill added to your diet can help prevent this.

Is ketosis dangerous?

As long as your body has enough insulin, nutritional ketosis is safe for adults without chronic diseases and who are not pregnant. While in ketosis, a person can have normal blood sugar levels and not be in immediate danger. Women who are breastfeeding, trying to get pregnant, or already pregnant should avoid going into ketosis as it may reduce the amount of breast milk produced.

Additionally, it is not advised for those who are going through the following to eat for a state of ketosis:

- Pancreatitis
- Carnitine deficiency
- Liver failure
- Porphyria
- Disorders that affect the metabolism of dietary fat

Long-term ketosis can cause low blood sugar, fatty liver, fatigue, chronic constipation, elevated cholesterol levels, and an increased risk of kidney stones in certain persons, although this is not guaranteed. Always talk to your doctor before starting any new eating regimen.

Can a diabetic person enter ketosis without being in ketoacidosis?

Yes! Many people with diabetes follow a ketogenic diet and remain in ketosis while maintaining a normal blood sugar range, even though you should always consult your doctor before starting any new eating plan. In fact, several studies confirm the advantages of a ketogenic diet and maintaining ketosis for those with diabetes. People with diabetes who followed the ketogenic diet dropped an average of 26 pounds, according to two-year research. According to separate research, the ketogenic diet increased people's insulin sensitivity by 75%. Staying in ketosis with a very low carbohydrate diet has even been shown to reduce hba1c levels in patients with diabetes if practiced for three months or longer.

Always talk to your doctor before changing your diet or medicines because being on a ketogenic diet and/or entering ketosis might impact how much insulin and/or diabetic medication you need.

The key difference between ketosis and ketoacidosis

While the body produces ketones in both conditions, the mechanisms behind the production of ketones differ between ketosis and ketoacidosis.

Ketoacidosis, a very severe condition brought on by ketones and inadequate insulin, can result in a diabetic coma or even death if untreated. It usually only affects those with insulin-dependent diabetes, although people with other forms of diabetes, an overactive thyroid, malnutrition, or alcoholism can also develop the condition.

On the other hand, the ketones produced by the body in a state of ketosis come about as a result of the body utilizing fat as fuel rather than carbs, frequently as a result of fasting or eating a very low carbohydrate diet. If you have diabetes and are interested in learning how to enter ketosis, consult your doctor before making any dietary or pharmaceutical modifications.

What to Eat and Avoid on a Low-Carb Diet

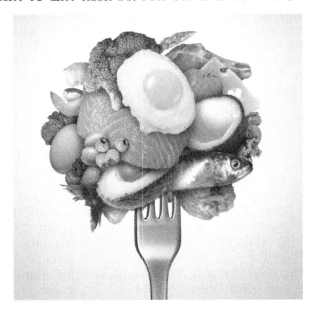

It might be difficult to initially stick to a low-carb, healthy diet, especially if you're new to it. After you understand a few basic guidelines, you'll be astonished at how simple it is to follow the keto diet. Whether your objective is to treat a health issue like type 2 diabetes, Parkinson's, Alzheimer's, insulin resistance, or epilepsy or to lose weight, this fast guide to keto-friendly foods can help you make the best choices.

Which Foods Should I Eat on a Keto Diet?

KetoDiet is about changing to a better lifestyle rather than merely trying to lose weight as quickly as possible. Contrary to popular belief, the ketogenic diet is not centered around cheese, bacon, and eggs. No matter how few carbohydrates there are, you should prioritize actual food and pay attention to its quality. Various whole foods, such as meat, fish, seafood, eggs, vegetables, nuts, full-fat dairy, and occasionally some fruit, such as berries, should be a part of a well-planned ketogenic diet.

Which Foods Should I Avoid on a Keto Diet?

Your daily carbohydrate restriction on a traditional ketogenic diet will be 20 to 25 grams of net carbohydrates (or 30 to 50 grams of total carbs).

Thus, you must avoid all high-carb items, such as grains (such as cereal, pasta, rice, and bread), potatoes, most legumes, sugar, and fruits. Additionally, processed meals and inflammatory fats should be avoided or consumed in moderation. A low-carb diet is simple to follow on our KetoDiet App. You'll discover hundreds of low-carb recipes, how-to articles, expert advice, and daily monitoring – everything you need to follow a healthy keto diet in one place.

The most popular low-carb foods suggested for the ketogenic diet are listed in detail below.

EAT Freely:

- Grass-fed and wild animal sources: Grass-fed meat (goat, venison, beef, lamb), ghee, wild-caught fish and seafood (avoid farmed fish), pastured eggs, gelatin, pastured pork and poultry, and butter - these are high in healthy omega-3 fatty acids (avoid meat covered in breadcrumbs and sausages, hot dogs, meat that comes with starchy or sugary sauces), offal, grass-fed (kidneys, liver, heart, and other organ meats)
- Healthy fats: Saturated fats (chicken fat, duck fat, lard, tallow, clarified butter (ghee), butter, goose fat, MCT oil, and coconut oil)

- Monounsaturated fats: (macadamia oil, olive oil, and avocado oil)
- Polyunsaturated fats: omega-3 fatty acids, especially from animal sources (fatty fish and seafood)
- Non-starchy vegetables and mushrooms: Leafy greens (Spinach, lettuce, swiss chard, bok choy, radicchio, chard, chives, endive, etc.). Some cruciferous vegetables like kohlrabi, kale (dark leaf), radishes. Celery stalk, summer squash (spaghetti squash, zucchini), asparagus, cucumber, bamboo shoots. Mushrooms (Portobello, shiitake, white, brow, chanterelle, etc.)
- Fruits: olives, avocado, coconut
- Beverages and Condiments: Coffee (black or with coconut milk or cream), water (still), tea (herbal, black)
- Pork rinds (cracklings) for "breading"
- Pesto, bone broth (make your own), pickles, mayonnaise, mustard, fermented foods (kombucha, kimchi, and sauerkraut (make your own)
- All herbs and spices, lime or lemon juice, and zest
- Whey protein (beware of artificial sweeteners, additives, soy lecithin, and hormones), egg white protein, and gelatin (hormone-free, grass-fed)

EAT Occasionally:

- Vegetables and Fruits: Some cruciferous vegetables (green and white cabbage, broccoli, turnips, brussels sprouts, red cabbage, cauliflower, fennel, swede/ rutabaga). Nightshades (tomatoes, peppers, eggplant). Some root vegetables (parsley root), leek, onion, spring onion, winter squash (pumpkin), garlic. Sea vegetables (homburg, nori), okra, sugar snap peas, bean sprouts, globe or French artichokes, wax beans, water chestnuts. Berries (blueberries, blackberries, strawberries, mulberries, raspberries, cranberries, etc.)
- Grain-fed animal sources and full-fat: Dairy Poultry, beef, ghee, and eggs (avoid farmed pork, it is too high in omega-6 fatty acids). Dairy products (cottage cheese, plain full-fat yogurt, sour cream, cheese, heavy cream) - avoid products labeled "low-fat" because most of them are packed with starch and sugar that will only stimulate your appetite.
- Bacon: beware of added starches (nitrates are acceptable if you consume foods high in antioxidants) and preservatives

- Nuts and seeds: Macadamia nuts (high in monounsaturated fats, very low in carbs). Walnuts, hazelnuts, pecans, almonds, pine nuts, sesame seeds, sunflower seeds, flaxseed, pumpkin seeds, chia seeds, hemp seeds. Brazil nuts (beware of high levels of selenium – do not consume too many of them!)
- Fermented soy products: If eaten, only non-GMO and fermented soy products such as tamari (gluten-free soy sauce), paleo-friendly coconut aminos, or Natto, Tempeh. Edamame (green soy beans), black soybeans – unprocessed
- Condiments: healthy zero-carb sweeteners (Swerve, Stevia, Erythritol, etc.). Thickeners: xanthan gum (xanthan gum isn't paleo-friendly - some people following the paleo diet use it, as you only need little amount), arrowroot powder. Sugar-free tomato products (passata, puree, ketchup). Carob and cocoa powder, extra dark chocolate (more than 70 percent, better 90 percent, and beware of soy lecithin). Beware of sugar-free mints and chewing gums - some of them have carbs from sugar alcohols like xylitol, sorbitol, and maltitol that may increase blood sugar and cause digestive problems
- Some Fruits, Vegetables, Seeds, and Nuts with Average Carbohydrates: based on your daily carb limit
- Root vegetables: beetroot, parsnip, celery root, carrot, and sweet potato
- Watermelon, Galia / Cantaloupe / Honeydew melons
- Cashew nuts and pistachio, chestnuts

Only very little amounts, better avoided completely:
- Dragon fruit (Pitaya), apricot, peach, grapefruit, kiwifruit, nectarine, apple, kiwi berries, cherries, pears, orange, plums, figs (fresh)
- Alcohol: Dry white wine, spirits (unsweetened), dry red wine - avoid for weight loss, only for weight maintenance.

Avoid Completely:
- Food rich in factory-farmed meat, carbohydrates, and processed foods
- Foods with added sugar. Avoid sweeteners that increase blood sugar, stimulate your appetite, cause insulin spikes and kick you out of ketosis.

- All grains, even whole meals (oats, corn, wheat, rye, barley, sorghum, rice, amaranth, millet, bulgur, sprouted grains, buckwheat), white potatoes, and quinoa. This includes all products made from grains (pizza, cookies, pasta, bread, crackers, etc.), sugar, and sweets (HFCS, agave syrup, cakes, table sugar, ice creams, sugary soft drinks, and sweet puddings).
- Factory-farmed fish and pork are high in inflammatory omega-6 fatty acids. Farmed fish may contain PCBs; avoid fish high in mercury.
- Processed foods containing carrageenan (e.g., almond milk products - watch for additives), BPAs (they do not have to be labeled!), MSG (e.g., in some whey protein products), wheat gluten, sulphites (e.g., gelatin, dried fruits).
- Artificial sweeteners (Equal sweeteners containing Aspartame, Splenda, Acesulfame, Saccharin, Sucralose, etc.) may cause cravings and have also been associated with other health issues such as migraines.
- Refined fats/oils (e.g., cottonseed, canola, sunflower, safflower, soybean, corn oil, grapeseed), trans fats such as margarine.
- Low-carb," "zero-carb," and "Low-fat" products (diet soda and drinks, Atkins products, mints, and chewing gums may be high in carbs or contain gluten, artificial additives, etc.)
- Milk (only small amounts of raw, full-fat milk is allowed). Milk isn't recommended for several reasons. Firstly, milk is difficult to digest because it lacks the "good" bacteria (eliminated through pasteurization) and may contain hormones. Secondly, it's rich in carbs (4-5 grams per 100 ml). For tea and coffee, replace milk with cream in reasonable amounts. You may have a small amount of raw milk but watch for the added carbohydrates. Lastly, American farmers utilize genetically modified bovine growth hormone (rBGH). Dairy cows are given rBGH injections to boost milk production. Choose full-fat dairy products labeled "NO rBGH."
- Alcoholic, sweet drinks (sweet wine, beer, cocktails, etc.)

- Tropical fruit (banana, papaya, pineapple, mango, etc.) and high-carb fruit (grapes, tangerine, etc.) Also, avoid fruit juices (including 100 percent fresh juices!) - It is preferable to drink smoothies, abut either way very limited. Smoothies contain fiber, which is at least more satiating than juices, which are sugary water. This also includes dried fruit (raisins, dates, etc.).

- Avoid soy products primarily for health concerns, aside from a few non-GMO fermented products, which are renowned for their health advantages. Likewise, stay away from any wheat gluten that may be present in low-carb dishes. You should not eat any part of bread when you give up bread. Avoid BPA-lined cans. Use glass jars or other naturally BPA-free containers wherever you can, or create your ketchup, coconut milk, ghee, or mayonnaise. BPA has been linked to several harmful health effects, including cancer and impaired thyroid function. Other additives to stay away from includes: MSG (present in some whey protein products) (e.g., in dried fruits, gelatin), carrageenan (e.g., almond milk products), and sulfites (e.g., in gelatin, dried fruits)

- Legumes (lentils, peanuts, beans, chickpeas, etc.). Legumes, except peanuts, have a fair amount of carbohydrates and should be avoided. Legumes are difficult to digest due to lectins and phytates, in addition to their high carbohydrate content. They have been linked to Hashimoto's, PCOS, IBS, and leaky gut syndrome. Some people steer clear of peanuts, while others consume them in moderation

Benefits

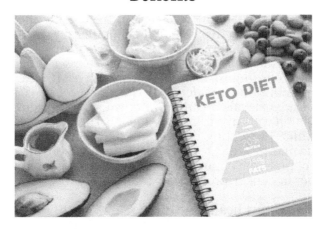

The diet works by reducing the body's supply of sugar. It will consequently start to breakdown fat for energy. As a result, the body produces molecules known as ketones, which it uses as fuel. When the body burns fats, it can lead to weight loss. The Standard Ketogenic Diet and the Cyclical Ketogenic Diet are two of the several forms of keto diets.

In this chapter, we explain the benefits and risks of the keto diet.

1. Supports weight loss

The ketogenic diet can aid in weight loss. Ketogenic diets consist of foods that may lower hunger-stimulating hormones. For these reasons, following a ketogenic diet may decrease hunger and aid in weight reduction. According to Trusted Source of 13 different randomized controlled studies, those on ketogenic diets lost 2 pounds (lbs) more over a year than those on low-fat diets. Similarly, another review of 11 studies revealed that after 6 months, those who followed a ketogenic diet lost 5 more pounds than those who adopted low-fat diets.

2. Improves acne

Acne has different causes and may be linked to some people's blood sugar and diet. Eating a diet rich in refined and processed carbohydrates may change the balance of gut bacteria and create major swings in blood sugar, both of which can harm the skin's health. According to 2012 research, a ketogenic diet could help some people with acne symptoms by reducing carbohydrate intake.

3. Might lower the risk of some cancers

Researchers have looked at how the ketogenic diet could be used to cure or possibly prevent some types of cancer. According to one study, certain cancer patients may benefit from using the ketogenic diet as a safe and effective supplemental therapy in addition to chemotherapy and radiation therapy. This is because it would kill cancer cells by inducing greater oxidative stress in them than in normal cells. According to a recent study from 2018, the ketogenic diet may minimize the incidence of insulin problems because it lowers blood sugar levels. Insulin is a hormone that regulates blood sugar and may have links to some cancers. The ketogenic diet may have some value in treating cancer, but according to some studies, there aren't many studies in this area. Additional research is required to completely comprehend the potential advantages of the ketogenic diet in cancer prevention and therapy.

4. May improve heart health

When following the ketogenic diet, making healthy meal selections is crucial. According to some research, consuming healthy fats like avocados instead of unhealthy fats like pork rinds can help lower cholesterol and improve heart health. According to a 2017 review of studies on animals and humans, the levels of total cholesterol, low-density lipoprotein (LDL), or "bad" cholesterol, and triglycerides in some people on the ketogenic diet significantly decreased, while levels of high-density lipoprotein (HDL), or "good" cholesterol, increased. Cardiovascular disease risk can rise with high cholesterol levels. Because a keto diet lowers cholesterol, it may lessen a person's chance of developing cardiac problems.

The research did come to the conclusion that the quality of the food is what determines how well the diet affects heart health. As a result, it's critical to consume a diet that is nutritionally balanced and healthy.

5. May protect brain function

According to some research, including this 2019 review, the ketones produced by the ketogenic diet may have neuroprotective benefits, which means they help support and protect the nerve cells and the brain.

Due to this, a ketogenic diet may aid in managing or preventing conditions like Alzheimer's disease. However, further study is required to determine how a ketogenic diet affects the brain.

6. Potentially reduces seizures

The keto diet modifies how the body consumes energy and causes ketosis due to the proportions of fat, protein, and carbohydrates.

The metabolic state of ketosis occurs when the body burns ketone bodies as fuel. According to the Epilepsy Foundation, ketosis can lessen seizures in epilepsy patients, particularly those who have not responded to conventional forms of therapy. This appears to work best on kids with focal seizures, but further study is needed to determine its effectiveness. A 2019 review supports that persons with epilepsy can benefit from a ketogenic diet. The ketogenic diet may lessen the symptoms of epilepsy through several different processes.

7. Improves PCOS symptoms
A hormonal condition known as polycystic ovary syndrome (PCOS) can cause an excess of male hormones, ovulatory failure, and polycystic ovaries. A high-carbohydrate diet can negatively affect those with PCOS, such as weight gain and skin issues. The ketogenic diet and PCOS have not been the subject of many clinical investigations.

Five women were studied in one pilot research over 24 weeks in 2005. The researchers discovered that a ketogenic diet improved several PCOS markers, including:

- hormone balance
- weight loss
- levels of fasting insulin
- follicle-stimulating hormone (FSH) and ratios of luteinizing hormone (LH)

A different review of studies from 2019 discovered that patients with hormonal abnormalities, such as PCOS and type 2 diabetes, benefited from a ketogenic diet. They did, however, add a warning that the research were too diverse to suggest a ketogenic diet as a general PCOS treatment.

Risks And Complications

The ketogenic diet may have a range of health benefits. Long-term adherence to the ketogenic diet, however, may have negative health effects, including an elevated risk of the following conditions:
- excess protein in the blood
- kidney stones
- vitamin and mineral deficiencies
- a build-up of fat in the liver

Many individuals refer to the negative side effects of the ketogenic diet as "keto flu." These negative outcomes may include:

- Constipation
- Low blood sugar
- Fatigue
- Nausea
- Headaches
- Low tolerance for exercise
- Vomiting

The keto diet should be avoided by some populations, including:

- Those with diabetes who are insulin-dependent
- Those who have eating disorders
- People who have pancreatitis or renal disease
- Women who are pregnant or breastfeeding

A ketogenic diet should not be adopted by people who use sodium-glucose cotransporter 2 (SGLT2) inhibitors, a form of medicine for type 2 diabetes. This medication raises the risk of diabetic ketoacidosis, a severe condition that increases acidity in the blood.

Any proposed diet plan should be discussed with a doctor, dietician, or other qualified healthcare professional, especially if the person is trying to manage a health problem or disease. To make sure the keto diet is a safe eating pattern, those thinking about starting it should visit a doctor and disclose any existing medical concerns, such as diabetes, heart disease, hypoglycemia, or other diseases.

Remember that there isn't enough research on the long-term advantages of the ketogenic diet. It is unclear if following this diet for longer periods is more beneficial than following less strenuous healthy eating habits.

Carbs are severely restricted on a ketogenic diet. Some carbs do, however, provide health benefits. People should eat a variety of nutrient-dense, fiber carbohydrates, such as fruits and vegetables, with wholesome protein sources, and healthy fats for a less restricted diet.

CHAPTER 2

What Happens To Women's Bodies After 60

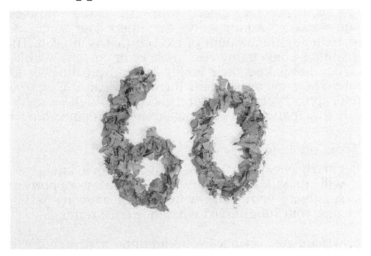

Long life is a blessing that some never get to experience. But for those who do, that blessing is accompanied by certain inescapable aging symptoms. Your body changes as you age, which is not always bad; it's simply different. Understanding what to expect can help you welcome these changes and alert you to what you can do to speed up the process. While some of these changes may be gradual and subtle, others may appear to occur suddenly. No matter when they occur, it's critical to understand that they're normal.

Ways Your Body Changes As You Age
Cardiovascular System: Your heart and blood arteries grow more inflexible as you age, and the heart fills with blood less quickly. The more inflexible the arteries are, the less room they have to expand as blood is pushed through them, which is why older persons are more likely to develop high blood pressure. A healthy older heart still functions normally, but it simply cannot pump as much blood or at the same rate as a younger heart. Because of this, older athletes often don't perform as well as younger ones. The death rate from heart-related disorders has decreased due to the numerous medical advancements accomplished during the past 20 years.

As you age, your heart and arteries get more rigid; therefore, it's critical to take all reasonable steps to maintain the health of your cardiovascular system. A nutritious diet and physical activity, particularly aerobic exercise, are two excellent ways to accomplish this.

Lungs: As you become older, your rib cage's muscles and diaphragm weaken. Additionally, the lungs lose some of their elasticity, reducing the amount of oxygen that is inhaled. This can make breathing challenging for smokers or anyone with a lung disease. Your lungs lose their ability to fend off illnesses as they deteriorate. These bacteria might linger and cause issues because they cannot spread germs without a good stiff cough.
The two best activities you can engage in to enhance lung health are:

- Avoid smoking
- Regularly engage in aerobic activity of some kind.

Exercise will provide your lungs the greatest opportunity to continue supplying your body with oxygen allowing you to stay active because your lungs aren't what they once were.

Immune System: As you age, your immune system becomes less effective. According to MedilinePlus, this may result in the following issues:

- Your immune system tends to react to stimuli more slowly, raising your risk of getting sick.
- Vaccines like those for the flu and pneumonia could not be as effective or durable as they once were.
- Because you have fewer immune cells as you age, your body recovers itself more slowly.
- You have a higher chance of getting cancer because as you become older, your body becomes less capable of identifying and repairing cell flaws.

An autoimmune illness is one where your immune system unintentionally targets and kills healthy bodily tissue. It's essential to take good care of yourself to help you keep your immune system as strong as possible. Get the vaccines your doctor advises, such as those for pneumonia, shingles, pneumococcal disease, and the flu (you can receive a high-dose flu vaccine starting at age 65). You can maintain a balanced diet, exercise, quit smoking, and consume less alcohol while building a robust immune system.

Urinary Tract: The urinary tract system often continues to function normally, barring any diseases or illnesses that affect it. If you're over 60, you've undoubtedly realized that you have to get up at least once throughout the night to use the bathroom. This is typical for this age group because as you get older, your bladder's capacity declines. Additionally, when the bladder muscles deteriorate, it may become harder to empty your bladder and shut the urinary sphincter, which might lead to leakage. These problems may lead to urinary incontinence. Some drugs can help with these issues, as well as pelvic floor (Kegel) exercises and bladder training.

Bones and Joints: Your bones and joints start to age beyond the age of 60. You absorb less calcium from your diet as you become older. Without calcium, your bones deteriorate and become brittle and feeble. Your body's ability to metabolize calcium is aided by vitamin D, which declines with age. Osteopenia (moderate loss of bone density) or osteoporosis may arise from a drop in calcium and vitamin D levels (severe loss of bone density). When osteoporosis appears, your chance of fracture and break increases significantly. Osteoporosis may be avoided by maintaining a healthy weight and engaging in weight-bearing exercises to promote bone density. You might want to discuss calcium and vitamin D supplements with your doctor.

Physical Changes As You Age

After many years of usage, your joints' surrounding cartilage may thin out, making movement painful. This cartilage deteriorates with time, making mobility difficult and perhaps dangerous. Osteoarthritis, a fairly common aging condition, may eventually develop from this. Unfortunately, wear and tear from years of usage causes joint discomfort, and surgery is now the only option to reverse it. Your doctor might occasionally recommend vitamins to aid with the discomfort. You might want to bring up this during your next appointment.

Muscle Tone and Body Fat: Around 30, your body begins to develop fat and lose muscle tone. The loss of muscle mass can be pretty substantial by the time you reach 60. According to MedilinePlus, only approximately 10 to 15% of muscle mass is lost as people age. The rest is a result of inactivity and a poor diet. The good news is that you can maintain or improve your muscle tone even after you become 60.

Ways Your Body Changes After You Turn 60

Strength training, often known as resistance training, is essential to maintaining and regaining muscular tone via regular exercise.

Eating healthily goes hand in hand with regular exercise. Together, these two substances can reduce body fat and improve muscular tone. With aging, body fat tends to rise. In this period of life, it's simple to develop a sedentary lifestyle as a habit. It's simple to develop the daily habit of doing virtually nothing, especially nothing physical because you become tired more quickly than you used to. Your chance of having diseases like diabetes is elevated by increased body fat. You can maintain a healthy body fat percentage by exercising regularly and eating a balanced diet.

Eyesight: You'll likely notice a difference in your vision by age 60. You could notice changes in your sense of color, a loss of close vision, and an increasing need for stronger lighting to read and discern details. These are generally caused by the lenses in your eyes stiffening and turning yellow. Your eyes may experience various physical changes as you age:

- Your eyes' whites can start to turn yellow.
- The whites of your eyes may develop a few specks of color.
- A gray-white ring may appear around the surface of the eye.
- Muscle loss may cause your lower lid to start drooping. If you lose fat around your eyes, it might make your eyes look sunken.

You'll probably notice as you get older that your eyes are often dry. To solve this issue, lubricating eye drops can be used. These changes to your eyes and vision are consequences of aging. See an eye doctor if they are painful or if you detect a significant change.

Hearing: Some hearing loss is not genuinely age-related; rather, it results from environmental exposure over time. Age-related hearing impairments, though, exist, such as the inability to perceive high-pitched noises. With aging, one's ability to detect high-pitched noises significantly decreases. Presbycusis is the name given to this age-related hearing loss. The ability to grasp what others are saying is the biggest problem with presbycusis. Consonants are difficult to hear because they are often uttered in a higher tone than vowels, caused by a mix of high-pitched voices, mainly those of women and children. Unfortunately, it ultimately gets harder to detect lower-pitched tones as well. Hearing difficulties might also result from earwax buildup and background noise. You can improve your hearing by maintaining clean ears and wearing hearing aids.

Teeth: As you reach 60, cavities become a major problem, mostly because of dry mouth. Dry mouth is not a problem exclusive to old age, but it is a side effect of many medications older people take for other illnesses. It's crucial to let your dentist know about any drugs you're taking so they may provide you with either an over-the-counter or a prescription treatment to assist battle the issue because a dry mouth can lead to cavities. Gum disease is another problem that frequently arises at any stage of life, especially as you age. While it is painless, if addressed, it can result in several issues, including tooth loss. After 60, mouth cancer becomes a risk as well. The average age of these patients is 62, and the American Cancer Society reports that 35,000 mouths, throat, and tongue cancer are detected yearly. Oral cancer typically has no discomfort in its early stages, and early identification can save lives. After age 60, your body will undergo physical changes. Your mouth, gums, and teeth can all benefit greatly from routine dental checkups. Early diagnosis saves money while also saving lives.

Skin: Your skin changes as you get older. It gets drier, thinner, less elastic, and more wrinkled.
Many things in the skin start to decrease, such as elastin, collagen, the layer of fat under the skin, nerve endings, sweat glands, blood vessels, and pigment-producing cells. The lack of these things causes your skin to become easily bruised and torn, sag and bag, crack and peel, and get age spots and wrinkles. A reduced sensitivity to discomfort also raises your risk of experiencing a heat stroke.

Body Changes After 50 and 60
You may be at risk for vitamin D insufficiency once you become 60 because your skin can no longer produce vitamin D from exposure to sunshine. If you want to prevent this problem, discuss taking a supplement with your doctor. Even while it's best to take care of your skin when you're young, there are still things you can do to protect it in the future. You can start using moisturizers and sunscreen, undergo surgical procedures like laser treatments, and your doctor may prescribe prescription drugs like hydroquinone for aging spots.

Accepting Physical Changes After 60
Aging is a privilege. Many people have remarked that they would have taken better care of their bodies if they had known they would live thus long. That sentence undoubtedly has a lot of truth for several people. While there is nothing you can do to change what you did or didn't do in the past, you can go forward and take the best possible care of yourself right now.

Practically all aspects of your evolving physique may be improved with regular exercise and a healthy diet. So stay active, eat healthily, and enjoy the rest of your life.

Why is Weight Loss After 60 Hard?

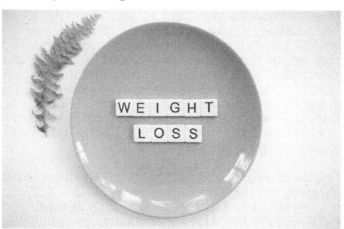

Let's face it; it isn't easy to lose weight after 60. You could eat whatever you wanted back in the day (for the most part). You consume a Hershey's Kiss and gain 2 pounds the next day. We lose the ability to consume anything we want as our bodies age. Suddenly, tracking calories and steps is necessary to beat weight. To understand why maintaining a healthy weight has suddenly become so challenging, read on for a list of 9 practical strategies to lose weight, remain in shape, and feel like you're 25 again.

Why Is Weight Loss So Difficult After 60?
Although many people begin to experience this annoyance around the age of 60, losing weight and keeping it off can become a problem as early as 50. What is happening?
Your metabolism is slowing down as a result of hormones. To begin with, as you become older, your metabolism decreases.

Robert Herbst on Losing Weight After 60: I'm 60; therefore, I understand what it is to be 60, says powerlifting expert and 19-time World Champion Robert Herbst. Loss of muscle mass results from decreased testosterone and human growth hormone (HGH) synthesis, which slows metabolism.

Carolyn Dean on Dieting After 60: Dr. Carolyn Dean, an author of 30 books, including The Complete Natural Medicine Guide to Women's Health, says, "Your efforts to lose weight are hampered because the loss of nutrients like magnesium has diminished the production of hormones that increase metabolism."

In essence, you are not to blame for this. Age-related declines in your body's ability to produce essential hormones make weight loss a challenge. Perimenopause and menopause are common conditions for women in their 50s and 60s. You burn fewer calories due to this change than you previously did.

Jill McKay on Over 60 Diet and Exercise: "Our body temperature would change during menstruation, which would result in an extra 300 calories burned each month, says Jill McKay, a certified personal trainer, and group fitness instructor. Although it's not much, over time, it adds up. Insulin resistance is a problem that occurs throughout both perimenopause and menopause and makes it increasingly harder to lose weight".

This means that you can no longer consume the foods you used to! This also applies to portions; you might discover that you can no longer consume as much as you formerly could without putting on weight.

You Have More Free Time to Socialize – And Eat!

There is more time when you are getting close to retirement. Of course, we would have more time to exercise, but is that really how we choose to spend our free time? Jill points out that elderly persons typically have greater possibilities for social interaction (and better finances to attend nice dinners). In fact, being among other eaters increases our propensity to eat more. It's challenging to maintain a healthy weight with all the socializing.

Potential Health Conditions to Be Aware Of

Most people find it difficult to lose weight beyond age 60, although this is normal. If, however, you are having difficulty losing weight, you might want to consult your doctor to ensure you are healthy.

The two most frequent medical problems that might result in weight gain are 1) the thyroid losing function and 2) insulin becoming less effective. If you can effectively metabolize your sugars, you can tell by the hemoglobin A1c test that is commonly administered. If not, diabetes could be a possibility for you.

These disorders are especially prevalent in women approaching menopause.

9 Practical Ways for Weight Loss After 60

So many men and women struggle with weight loss after age 60. To tip the scales in your favor, there are several techniques for shedding that weight.

1. Strength Training: Resistance training, often known as strength training, isn't typically the first exercise older adults choose. The most popular workouts are often cardio exercises like treadmill walking or elliptical.

Carol Michaels on healthy eating after 60

Carol Michaels, an Idea Fitness Trainer, is concerned that many seniors are overlooking the benefits of strength training. Strength training is often the exercise component that's missing in weight loss programs for those over 60. This workout strengthens and develops muscle using weights (or your body weight). It strengthens muscle fibers and fortifies tendons, bones, and ligaments. We lose muscle mass as we age, primarily due to our slowing metabolisms. This leads to an even slower metabolism, and before you know it, you're caught in a vicious cycle. Strength training, however, may break that pattern of muscle loss; it can reverse muscle loss at any age. "Muscle is metabolically active; therefore, the more muscle mass you have, the quicker your metabolism," Carol explains. Strength training can therefore aid with weight reduction.

But weight reduction is only one benefit of strength training. Additional advantages of strength training are:

- Better balance
- Less risk of injury
- Improved athletic performance
- Better agility
- Higher energy levels
- Better coordination

Another way to think about strength training, according to Robert Herbst, is that it causes the body to develop new muscle that is metabolically active and burns calories even while at rest.

This new muscle raises the metabolism, just like a six-cylinder car uses more fuel than a four-cylinder one, even when idling at a red light. Essentially, you've broken the vicious cycle of aging and begun a weight loss and control cycle. Your increased muscle will help you burn more fat.

DO I USE FREE WEIGHTS OR MACHINES?

Now that we are all in agreement that strength training is fantastic, you may ask how to do this. Many older adults, Carol claims, are in their mid-60s and have no idea where to start. Should you utilize the equipment at the gym? Do you need to purchase free weights? She continues, "While machines can be useful for people who have balance concerns, free weight exercise has several advantages. You can strength train at home with free weights and improve by one-pound increments. Using free weights teaches you how to move your body naturally throughout daily tasks. You can build more main muscle groups using free weights instead of a machine because you won't rely on them for support. Weight machines only work for large muscle groups. They can overlook the little but crucial stabilizer muscles that provide balance, coordination, and injury avoidance. Should I use machines or free weights in the gym or at home? Gyms offer free weights as well, so you have the option of purchasing your free weights or purchasing a gym membership.

DO I NEED TO STRENGTH TRAIN REGULARLY?

Strength training sounds great, but if you think I'm going to devote two hours a day to it, you're mistaken. Not to worry. You don't have to strength train like a madman to reap the rewards. Carol advises setting a goal of twice weekly. "Build up each muscle group, switching between your upper and lower body. To avoid creating imbalances, work the front, rear, and sides of the body. If you're over 60 and new to fitness, you could begin with a very light weight".

Strength training after 60

After you've scheduled your workouts, Carol advises performing the exercise 5–10 times. You should feel the muscle working around the fifth to eighth repetition. You should feel like you've exercised the muscle by the last repetition but not exhausted. If you are exhausted, you are doing too much weight. Many professionals online offer strength training plans with pictures and instructions, but you can call your local gym to have a personal trainer show you what exercises to do. Bodybuilding.com - do not be put off by the name - has a ton of pre-planned workout schedules. You can categorize them by length—4, 6, 8, 12 weeks, etc.—as well as by level—beginner, intermediate, and advanced.

2. Keep Carbs and Sugars Low

Even if you've never had a problem with delicious desserts and carb-heavy meals, dieting after 60 might be challenging because your body may start to change. Even if you've maintained your weight for years, that daily dessert can make you gain weight.

The larger issue, however, is that older persons over 60 have a propensity for increased blood sugar because of insulin resistance.

Denny Hemingson on Losing Weight After Age 60
Functional Diagnostic Nutrition Practitioner Denny Hemingson, 61, explains that insulin tells the liver, muscles, and fat cells to absorb glucose from the bloodstream. When such cells develop insulin resistance, glucose is not used and stays in the blood, leading to excessive blood sugar levels. Eventually, this leads to metabolic syndrome, type II diabetes, and pre-diabetes. In this situation, the body finds it considerably more difficult to shed additional pounds. The solution? Reducing carbohydrates. Denny continues by stating that it's crucial to focus on blood sugar retention in people over 60 and that cutting carbs will lower your blood sugar, making it easier to keep a healthy weight. The Keto diet, which has high fat, moderate protein, and low carbohydrate composition, is supported by Carolyn Dean. This enables the body to burn down its glycogen reserves of sugar from carbohydrates before activating fat burning to use the remaining fat cells as energy.

Although the Keto diet is steadily becoming more well-known in the health and fitness world as a means to burn fat more quickly than ever before, you are advised to see your doctor first. According to Carolyn, the Keto diet aims to limit your daily carb intake to 20–50 grams.

3. Drink Half Your Body Weight In Ounces of Water
Although drinking water doesn't in itself aid in weight loss, it's a fact that many individuals mistake thirst for hunger. The cure? Drink a ton of water. You should consume half your body weight (in lbs) in ounces of water, advise Carolyn and Denny. Carolyn says that people regularly mistakenly believe they are hungry when they are actually thirsty. So if you weigh 200 pounds, you must drink 100 ounces of water. That equates to 5–6 bottles of water each day.

4. Consider Adding Magnesium to Your Diet
You might not have considered including magnesium in your diet. Magnesium aids in synthesizing proteins, carbohydrates, and fats and boosts weight reduction and metabolism.

Carolyn notes that in the 700–800 magnesium-dependent enzymes, energy production is the most significant enzymatic reaction to which magnesium helps. Adenosine triphosphate (ATP), the primary energy storage molecule of the body, is activated by magnesium. You may easily add magnesium to your water to add it to your diet.

Add sea salt and an absorbable type of magnesium to your water, such as magnesium citrate powder, advises Carolyn. This will make sticking to a low-carb diet much simpler and prevent you from experiencing the energy loss, sluggishness, and headaches brought on by electrolyte loss. Another thing to consider is that since sugar depletes magnesium and strains the body, avoiding it can help counteract the effects of stress.

5. Get Some Sun
Don't get sunburn or anything, but please take vitamin D! If you don't get enough vitamin D, you might reach for more food than you need. Leptin and vitamin D work together to control hunger signals, according to Denny. This mechanism breaks down when vitamin D levels are low, which makes people overeat. You can get the Vitamin D you need by getting more sun. Go outside, enjoy the weather, and celebrate your ability to restrain your appetite!

6. Reduce Stress Through Yoga
It is well known that stress can make us overeat. When you're feeling stressed, do you reach for some chocolate ice cream from the freezer? You're not alone. Relaxing is an excellent approach to handling stress. And occasionally, you require some encouragement. Yoga, which does more than merely reduce stress, is suggested by Denny. Your balance, core strength, and awareness will all increase. Consider using meditation, prayer, and nature walks as additional stress-reduction techniques. The Simple Habit application includes free, brief meditations that you can try if you are interested in meditation.

7. Get Quality Sleep
The impact of sleep on your general health is incredible.
You will have greater energy for your strength training session, and your body also creates human growth hormones while you sleep (HGH). Denny suggests obtaining 7-8 hours of good sleep every night. The greatest way to ensure that you get a good night's sleep is to:

- Establish a regular bedtime habit by going to bed simultaneously every day.
- Avoid using a screen before bed (smartphones, computers, TVs).

So don't skimp on sleep—it keeps you young!

8. Consider Meal Prepping

Meal planning can make you eat healthier throughout the week, even when you don't have time to cook (or perhaps you're simply not in the mood). Stop consuming manufactured food, Jill advises. Yes, this is difficult if you live alone. Consider meal planning for the week so you can prepare larger portions and divide them into smaller meals throughout the week.

9. Don't Push Yourself Too Hard

Lastly, try not to be so hard on yourself. If a week passes without you dropping a pound, don't worry! That could be completely typical. According to our experts, you shouldn't drastically reduce your calorie consumption. Don't substantially reduce your calorie intake, Jill advises. "Adequate calories are vital! Muscle loss brought on by rapid weight reduction alters body composition and may impede metabolism. In other words, if you aren't eating enough, all of your strength training success might be undone. Last but not least, don't overwork yourself at the gym. Jill elaborates on her own pet peeve: "One of my biggest pet peeves is when an unskilled personal trainer attempts to force a Baby Boomer to do a workout that is so difficult that they are so sore the next day that they can hardly brush their teeth or get up off the toilet. That's not necessary at all! If you need a break, take one! If you feel the weight is too much, lighten up! The goal isn't to make yourself miserable but to maintain your health.

Ketogenic Diet And Menopause

Menopause is the stage when a woman's menstrual period ends for 12 months in a row. It signals the end of her reproductive and fertile years. Common side effects of changing hormone levels during menopause include mood changes, hot flashes, and sleep disruption. Following menopause, many women also suffer an average weight increase of roughly five pounds. Some people suggest the keto diet, which has a very low carbohydrate intake and a high-fat content, to reduce menopausal symptoms and maintain hormonal balance. However, because it might have unfavorable side effects, it might not be the ideal strategy for all women.

This chapter explores how several hormones might change while someone is in ketosis. It also looks at the possible advantages of this diet for menopausal women.

Keto and Hormones

Hormonal imbalances, particularly those involving estrogen and progesterone, can result during menopause. This can cause lower metabolism and decreased insulin sensitivity. Additionally, it could cause an increase in food cravings. There isn't much proof that the ketogenic diet can affect the ratio of reproductive hormones. However, the keto diet can significantly regulate the balance of certain hormones that affect insulin production and appetite management.

Benefits

Here are some potential benefits of the ketogenic diet for menopausal women.

Effect on Insulin Sensitivity: Insulin is a hormone that aids in transferring glucose (sugar) from your bloodstream into your cells to be utilized as an energy source. Hot flashes and night sweats, two symptoms of menopause, have also been shown to be significantly correlated with insulin resistance. Your body's cells develop insulin resistance when they don't react well to the hormone. This increases the amount of glucose circulating in your blood and increases your chance of developing a chronic disease. According to several research, the ketogenic diet may help persons with diabetes improve their insulin sensitivity, have lower insulin levels, and use fewer drugs to achieve their goal blood sugar levels. Additionally, one research tested the ketogenic diet on those with endometrial or ovarian cancer. According to the research, following the ketogenic diet for 12 weeks resulted in greater reductions in belly fat and increases in insulin sensitivity.

Effect on Weight Gain: People who are overweight or obese have been proven to benefit from the keto diet in terms of weight reduction, lipid profiles, and glycemic management. In one research, postmenopausal women examined four food regimens to determine which was most effective for maintaining weight. Researchers compared the Mediterranean diet to a low-fat, low-carb diet in line with the current Dietary Guidelines for Americans in the United States. At the study's conclusion, researchers discovered that those who consumed a diet low in carbohydrates, high in protein, and moderate in fat had a lower risk of weight gain. A low-fat diet, however, increased the likelihood of postmenopausal weight gain the most. It's crucial to note that the reduced-carb diet used in this study typically had 163 grams of carbs, which is significantly more than what is advised for a keto diet. There aren't many studies linking the ketogenic diet to menopausal-related weight gain.

Effect on Food Cravings: Many women report having more appetite and cravings throughout the menopausal transition and the postmenopausal years. It has been shown that the ketogenic diet increases feelings of fullness. For instance, one set of research indicates that being in ketosis may cause a decrease in hunger. This could be because of diets with a lot of protein and fat increase satiety through various mechanisms. This includes decreasing intestinal transit, decreasing gastric emptying, and playing a role in releasing hunger hormones. Another research examined 20 obese people to evaluate their dietary desires, sleep patterns, sexual activity, and general quality of life while adhering to a very low-calorie ketogenic diet. Researchers discovered that patients experienced improvements in their sexual function, good eating management, significant weight reduction, and overall quality of life.

Side Effects
The keto diet may offer some advantages for menopause, but it is not for everyone. The "keto flu" is a common group of side effects that you may experience after beginning the keto diet. This is because switching to a very low carbohydrate diet requires some time for your body to adjust.

The following symptoms are linked to the keto flu:

- Brain fog
- Headache
- Body aches
- Feeling faint
- Stomach pain/discomfort
- Dizziness
- Sore throat
- Flu-like symptoms
- Fatigue
- Nausea
- Heartbeat changes

When the diet is carefully followed, symptoms often peak in the first week and progressively subside during the next three weeks. The negative effects that the keto diet could have on your general heart health are another issue. A few studies have suggested that a ketogenic diet's high quantities of saturated fat might raise the levels of low-density lipoprotein (LDL), or bad cholesterol, in our bodies.

Diets high in fat have also been linked with inflammation and the disruption of gut microbiota (bacteria in the digestive system). Additionally, some people are concerned about the rigorous restriction on carbs, usually less than 50 grams. This is so because many items high in carbohydrates prohibited by the keto diet are also high in nutrients, including fiber, vitamins, and minerals. If you don't take the right supplements, you might be at risk for vitamin shortages. Menopause may be frustrating and difficult for some women, as can the time immediately after menopause. Know that you are not alone. Menopause-related weight gain can be lessened by adopting good eating habits and frequent exercise routines. Although the keto diet may help some people's symptoms, it's not a one-size-fits-all solution. Finding out which eating strategy will work best for you requires a conversation with your healthcare physician and a qualified dietitian.

Mistakes Beginners Make and How to Avoid Them

Given the paucity of data on the ketogenic diet, it might be difficult to predict whether or not you will have any specific effects, such as weight reduction. It can be challenging to follow the keto diet "properly" because it is so severely restrictive. For instance, you'll have to forgo starchy vegetables, limit fruits, and avoid grains, sauces, juice, and sweets on this diet. Moreover, as per the standard keto food list, you must consume a lot of fats (lots of them). By doing this, you'll enter the metabolic state of ketosis, which causes your body to burn fat instead of carbs, potentially increasing your weight loss. However, because fats exist in various forms (not all healthy) and carbohydrates are present in almost everything, it may be easy to err here, especially if you're new to the keto diet.
To ensure you're using this technique as safely as possible, avoid the following common keto pitfalls:

1. Cutting Your Carbs and Increasing Your Fat Too Much Too Quickly_ You might be eating cereal, sandwiches, and spaghetti one day and then decide to start the keto diet and limit your daily carbohydrate intake to 20 grams (g), which is usually the suggested starting point. (For reference, a medium apple provides 25 g of carbohydrates.) That can be a major adjustment for your body. Consider easing in. According to Lara Clevenger, a ketogenic dietitian-nutritionist, "before starting a keto diet, individuals may benefit from weaning down their carbohydrate consumption instead of reducing carbohydrates cold turkey."

2. Not Drinking Enough Water on Keto: For all the attention on what you are eating, don't overlook what you're drinking. On a ketogenic diet, dehydration is more likely to occur. "Your fluid and electrolyte balance may change due to the ketogenic diet's significant reduction in carbohydrate intake".

According to Alyssa Tucci, RDN, nutrition manager at Virtual Health Partners in New York City, "carbs are stored in the body together with water, so when these reserves are depleted, that water is lost along with them. She further claims that the removal of the accumulated ketones in urine by the body depletes it of salt and water. All that to say: Drink up. All of this to say: Cheers! To meet the recommendation of drinking half your body weight in ounces of water each day, Tucci advises waking up to a large glass of water and sipping on it frequently throughout the day.

3. Failing to prepare for the keto flu: During the first two weeks of the keto diet, you may suffer what is known as the "keto flu," or flu-like symptoms (such as muscular cramps, nausea, pains, and exhaustion), as your body switches from being a carbohydrate burner to a fat burner. Please note that not everyone experiences it. If you're not ready for this feeling, you could assume something is wrong and stop your diet altogether. More than that, according to Clevenger, planning your meals or meal preparation can help you get through the low-energy phase of the transition. She also suggests drinking plenty of water, consuming meals high in potassium, magnesium, and sodium, and other measures to deal with keto flu symptoms.

4. Forgetting to Consume Omega-3 Fatty Acid-Rich Foods: Don't limit yourself to bacon, cheese, and cream, even if fat is the main component of the diet. Aim to consume more anti-inflammatory omega-3 fatty acids, especially EPA and DHA, which are present in foods like salmon, herring, sardines, oysters, and mussels, adds Clevenger. (If seafood isn't your thing, try krill oil or cod liver oil.) If you haven't loaded up on avocado, olive oil, and seeds like chia and flaxseed, do so. Other healthy fats are also a wonderful option. Not only are they keto-friendly, but they also provide the beneficial polyunsaturated and monounsaturated fats your body needs to function at its peak.

5. Not adding enough salt to your food: Given that people consume more sodium than ever in a diet high in processed foods, you probably aren't used to hearing the recommendation to consume more salt. However, it's essential for keto.

Not only does the body lose sodium when ketones are cleared from the body, but you may also consume significantly less table salt now that you've eliminated the main source of salt in the typical American diet: packaged, processed foods like bread, crackers, cookies, and chips. Table salt is made up of 40% sodium and 60% chloride.

"If you're on a ketogenic diet, chances are you'll need to make most, if not all, of your meals and snacks from scratch, so simply season with salt," Tucci advises.

6. Going It Alone and Not Clearing the Diet With Your Doc: Many people try the ketogenic diet, hoping it will treat a medical condition. If that is you, Clevenger advises that you first consult your physician to get their approval of your plan, particularly if you are also on medication. As your signs and symptoms improve, your doctor may need to change certain drugs," she adds. An example is insulin, which may require a lower dosage given your strict carbohydrate restriction.

7. Ignoring your intake of vegetables: Veggies contain carbs. You must thus be careful with how much food you consume, even lettuce. You risk consuming too many carbohydrates if you're careless or eating them randomly, which will cause you to exit ketosis. On the other hand, if keeping track of every small carrot becomes too challenging, you may skip vegetables altogether. But while watching amounts and properly tracking carbohydrates, it's vital to include veggies because they contain fiber that helps avoid constipation, a possible side effect of the keto diet. Choose nonstarchy foods in a rainbow of colors for a range of nutrients, advises Tucci, like leafy greens, broccoli, cauliflower, cucumber, tomato, asparagus, and bell peppers.

8. Getting Obsessed with Carb Counting and Ignoring the Importance of Food Quality: When significantly reducing carbohydrates seems to be the only purpose of the keto diet, everything else may seem like an afterthought. "Reducing your carbohydrate consumption is important, but when finances allow, focusing on higher-quality items can help enhance your health, too," claims Clevenger. This entails choosing foods high in omega 3, such as wild salmon, organic meats, or grass-fed, local, and choosing whole foods for snacks rather than prepared keto-friendly items. It also involves including as many nutrient-dense fruits and vegetables in your diet as you can to maintain a balanced diet. Many qualified dietitians aren't fans of the keto diet because it could result in dietary deficits. You can prevent these by working with an RD personally as you follow the keto diet.

CHAPTER 3

Keto And Exercise

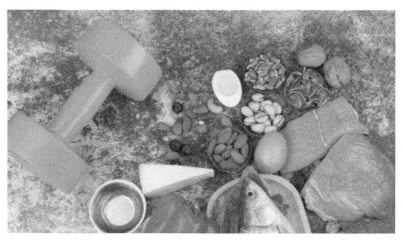

Before you begin combining keto with exercise, there are a few key points that experts want you to be aware of. You've heard of the ketogenic (also known as the keto) diet by now; you know, the one that pushes you to consume a lot of healthy fats while largely avoiding carbohydrates. The keto diet has entered the mainstream and is especially well-liked by the fitness crowd. It was formerly used to treat people with epilepsy and other significant health conditions. While it's true that it may have some performance advantages, doctors say there are certain crucial facts you should be aware of if you're considering going out while on the ketogenic diet.

At first, you might not feel so great. Naturally, not feeling your best might affect your workouts. Ramsey Bergeron, a keto athlete and NASM-certified personal trainer in Scottsdale, Arizona, says the first few days may seem like you're in a fog. "Your brain uses glucose (from carbohydrates) as its main energy source, so switching to ketone bodies produced by the liver's breakdown of fats would require some getting used to," he explains. Fortunately, the mental fog usually fades after a few days. Bergeron advises against exercising in dangerous situations that call for rapid reactions, such as riding a bike on the road with cars or taking a strenuous, prolonged outdoor hike. It's not a good idea to undertake a new workout during the first few weeks of a keto diet.

It's not a good idea to sign up for that new boot camp class you've wanted to take if you recently switched to a keto diet. Bergeron advises, "Keep doing what you are doing." This is mainly due to the first point: most people don't first feel great on keto. When extreme, this initial unpleasant phase—which typically passes within a few days to a couple of weeks—can be referred to as the "keto flu" due to its flu-like grogginess and gastrointestinal disturbances. However, it is probably not the time to try a new class or aim for a PR. "When my clients try anything new, I always advise them to keep the variables to a minimum," says Bergeron. "You won't know what worked and what didn't if you alter too many things at once," he continues.

It's essential that you eat enough before exercising while following a ketogenic diet.

"Make sure you're providing your body with enough energy, and avoid decreasing calories too strictly," advises Lisa Booth, R.D.N., a nutritionist and Nori Health's health lead. This is significant because, according to her, people on the keto diet tend to undereat. According to Booth, a keto diet also has an appetite-suppressing effect, so you can think you're not hungry even if you aren't providing your body with enough energy. "When you restrict an entire food category (in this case, carbohydrates), you often automatically decrease calories," she adds. You'll feel awful if you drastically cut calories while working out, which might affect your performance and results.

Low- and moderate-intensity workouts can help you burn more fat.

This is one of the key arguments favoring keto for weight reduction. "When you're in ketosis, you don't use glycogen as an energy source," says Booth. "Glycogen is a substance stored in muscles and tissues as a reserve of carbs. Instead, you're using ketone bodies and fat. A ketogenic diet can help enhance fat oxidation, spare glycogen, produce less lactate, and use less oxygen if you engage in aerobic workouts like biking or running," she clarifies. In other words, that may result in more fat being burnt during aerobic exercise. Booth continues, "But it probably won't improve performance". Furthermore, while following a ketogenic diet, you don't have to exert yourself to the fullest. According to Chelsea Axe, D.C., C.S.C.S., a certified strength, and conditioning specialist in Nashville, "Studies have indicated that ketogenic diets combined with moderate-intensity exercise can favorably impact one's body composition. Research has shown that ketogenic diets increase the body's capacity to burn fat both at rest and during low- to moderate-intensities, so your weight-loss efforts may be optimized when exercising in these zones," she says.

High-intensity exercises may be best avoided while on a diet.

According to Axe, studies have shown that diets heavy in a certain macronutrient, such as fat, encourage a greater capacity to use that macronutrient as fuel. However, she says, "regardless of your macronutrient ratio consumption, the body adjusts to using glycogen as fuel during high-intensity activity. You'll recall from earlier that carbs fuel glycogen stores, so if you don't consume a lot of them, your ability to execute higher-intensity exercise can be compromised. Instead, Axe argues that moderate exercise is best for maximizing the body's capacity to burn fat. As a result, those who participate in intense exercises like CrossFit or HIIT might benefit more from adopting a ketogenic diet during their off-season or when they are less concerned with their performance.

To profit from your workouts, you need to eat adequate fat.

This is essential; otherwise, you risk losing out on all the advantages and having your performance deteriorate. According to Bergeron, if you follow a ketogenic diet but don't consume enough fats, you are effectively following an Atkins diet with high protein, low carbs, and low fat. He says that doing so might make you incredibly hungry, reduce muscle mass, and be almost impossible to maintain. Most low-carb diets have a bad reputation for a reason. You're likely to experience fatigue and lose out on entering ketosis if you don't consume enough fat to make up for the carbs you're missing. According to Bergeron, most calories must come from good fat sources like fish, grass-fed meats, coconut oil, and avocado.

When combining diet with exercise, paying attention to your body is important.

This is true throughout your whole experience, but particularly in the first few weeks, you follow a ketogenic diet. According to Booth, "if you often feel tired, lightheaded, or drained, your body may not function properly on a very low-carb diet. "The most crucial factor should be your health and wellbeing. See how you feel after adding more carbohydrates. If this makes you feel better, the ketogenic diet might not be the best option for you," she suggests.

Keto-Friendly Drinks

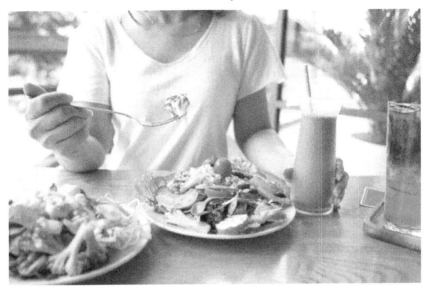

Yes, they exist.

What makes a drink keto?
Because the keto diet calls for getting fewer than 10% of your daily calories from carbs—roughly 20 to 30 grams a day—you should avoid drinks that exceed, or even better, fall well below, that percentage. Why? With very few exceptions, you don't want to consume all of your daily carbohydrate allowance in a single serving. When searching for keto-friendly options, look for beverages with less than 5 grams of carbohydrates on the nutrition label. Avoid heavily sweetened beverages (sorry, orange juice fans) or include additional sweeteners, which, regrettably, include most cocktails.

What beverages work best for a keto diet?
We searched for the most acclaimed and highly rated keto-friendly beverages for this list. Some choices are apparent (hello, number one), while others will have you rushing to Starbucks to get every keto-friendly beverage they offer. To ensure that you don't feel like you are missing out on anything, we have also provided several alcoholic alternatives and soda substitutes.

Before beginning the keto diet, consult a nutritionist and/or a doctor to ensure you're obtaining all the necessary nutrients. Do whatever seems right for you as well! All bodies are different.

Water

Yes, of course, we do. But water satisfies a keto-friendly substance's fundamental and most important condition: it contains little carbohydrates. Craig Clarke says on the keto site Ruled.me, "During the first few days of carbohydrate restriction, the body normally eliminates water and minerals at an accelerated pace. A few days later, when ketone levels rise, even more water than usual will be expelled." So drink up!

Sparkling Water

According to the aforementioned logcv, all zero-calorie seltzers are also keto. That means quitting your favorite La Croix habit won't be necessary if you go keto. The Sparkling Ice waters are also a favorite among many keto dieters. This Amazon reviewer wrote, "I'm on the keto diet and drink them constantly while still losing weight. They have a terrific flavor and satisfy my thirst. Additionally, each bottle has 0 calories and 0 or 5 carbohydrates."

Zevia Zero Calorie Soda

This keto-friendly Tiktok designer vouch for Zevia, saying, "If you are a soda-holic, Zevia is a wonderful solution to replace all that soda." Amazon shoppers adore it as a soda substitute because it contains neither calories nor sugar. Most diet sodas are also OK when following a ketogenic diet.

Green Tea

While on the keto diet, remember your body's other health requirements! Green tea adheres to the diet while providing much-needed antioxidants and minerals. Matcha powder is also included in this. According to Carine Claudepierre of the keto-focused SweetAsHoney blog, the ingredient comprises dried green tea leaves that have been crushed into green tea powder. It is carb-free and keto-friendly.

Black Tea

Black tea has no net carbohydrates, although heavy cream can be added for taste if desired, which is, in fact, keto-friendly. Tea is a good keto-friendly beverage because it's a perfect substitute for water and can be served hot or cold, according to the MunchMunchYum blog.

Bulletproof Coffee

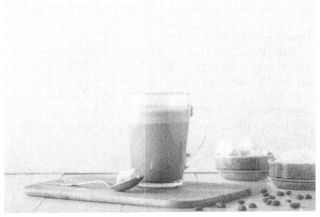

Yes, you can drink your coffee black, but adding that sweet, sweet (but low-carb, high-fat) butter can help you reach your calorie targets much more quickly. According to a blog article by WholesomeYum's Maya Krampf, "Bulletproof coffee is coffee brewed with either butter or ghee AND coconut oil or MCT oil. My favorite part is the extra energy I got from combining butter and MCT oil with my coffee. I usually feel satisfied after eating it and am attentive and productive."

Non-Dairy Milk Alternatives

Protein. Fat. Little carbohydrates. Everything is fine. Almond milk, according to Elana Amsterdam of Elana's Pantry, is the greatest milk for the keto diet. It has amazing flavor and mouthfeel and is relatively low in carbohydrates, making it my favorite."

Protein Shakes
Now that everyone is interested in going keto, several protein powders are made expressly for the keto diet. You may either make your own or choose an Atkins-style shake. It has almost 23,000 five-star ratings on Amazon, and one reviewer claimed that it doesn't taste like "a 'diet' item". "I use this to satisfy my weet tooth craving while on the keto diet."

Hard Liquor
The blog Green and Keto claimed that "alcohols like vodka, scotch, rum, whiskey, gin, and tequila are great options on the keto diet. They have no carbohydrates or sugar when eaten alone". Just be careful not to combine them with any liquids or calorie sweeteners.

Your best friends in keto mixers are sugar-free sodas, seltzers, and tonics.

Starbucks' Peach Citrus White Tea
After the drink became quite popular, there was considerable disagreement about whether it was keto-friendly, but in reality, it is. Only Starbucks' unsweetened Peach Citrus White Tea, heavy cream, two to four pumps of sugar-free vanilla syrup, and ice are combined to make it. All of those things are in the (keto) clear. A few low-carb blogs have even created versions of their recipes you can make at home.

Starbucks Pink Drink
The OG Pink Drink wasn't originally keto, but early adopters of the diet quickly figured out how to make it such.
To give this drink a keto makeover, request a sugar-free syrup, unsweetened Passion Tango tea, and light or heavy creamer. "Grammable keto," boom. This TikTok creator said, "It is one of my favorite clean keto Starbucks beverages.

Lagunitas Daytime IPA
This beer has an ABV of 4%, fewer than 100 calories, and 3 grams carbohydrates. This indicates that it is keto-friendly, and the designer of the keto Tiktok claims that it has a "cool name" and "tastes amazing."

Michelob Ultra Beer
"Michelob Ultra is below 3 g carbs per serving and has 95 calories," Joe Duff of The Diet Chef wrote in a blog post. "It has a refreshing flavor with a little bit of sweetness."

CHAPTER 4

Recipes

Breakfast

1. Banana Keto Chia Pudding

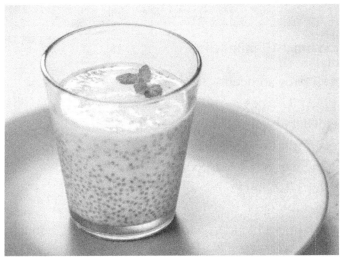

Servings: 1
Preparation time: 130 minutes
Ingredients
- White Yoghurt - 2 tablespoons
- Chia seeds - 1, 5 tbsp
- KetoDiet protein drink banana flavor - 1
- Milk - 150 ml

Instructions
Mix all the ingredients together, pour the mixture into a glass and let it solidify in the refrigerator for at least 2 hours. Decorate with a sprig of mint, for example.

2. Green Keto Smoothie

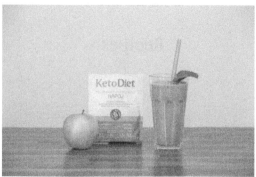

Servings: 1
Preparation time: 15 minutes
Ingredients

- Fresh baby spinach - 30 g
- Apple - 1/2 pcs
- KetoDiet Protein Drink - 1 serving
- Coconut milk - 200 ml
- Young barley - 1 teaspoon
- Water - 100 ml

Instructions
Pour the milk into a blender, add sliced apple, baby spinach, water, protein drink, and young barley and mix all the ingredients thoroughly. Garnish the smoothie with a slice of lemon and serve.

3. Matcha Keto Pudding

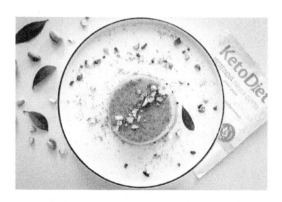

Servings: 1
Preparations: 60 minutes
Ingredients

- Matcha tea - 1 teaspoon
- Chia seeds - 20 g
- KetoDiet protein panna cotta - 1 serving
- Almond milk - 100 ml
- Nuts mix for decoration
- Vanilla essence according to taste

Instructions
Mix the powder from the protein panny cotty bag and matcha tea into the almond milk, add the chia seeds, and mix the vanilla essence. Pour into a bowl and let it solidify in the refrigerator for at least 45 minutes. Garnish the protein matcha pudding with chopped nuts and serve.

4. Keto Waffles with Chocolate Cottage Cheese

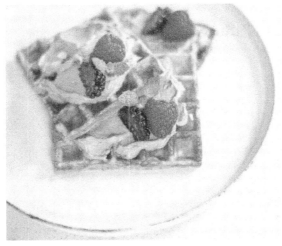

Servings: 2
Preparation time: 30 minutes
Ingredients

- Cocoa - 1 tbsp
- KetoDiet Protein drink hazelnut flavor and chocolate - 1 tbsp
- KetoDiet Protein drink creamy without flavor - 2 measuring cups

- Baking powder - 1/4 teaspoon
- Almond flour - 30 g
- Butter - 40 g
- Milk - 120 ml
- Whole cottage cheese - 1 piece
- Cinnamon - 1/2 teaspoon
- Vanilla essence according to taste
- Egg - 2 pcs

Instructions

Prepare the dough for 6 waffles. In a bowl, mix almond flour, KetoDiet protein powder, baking powder, cinnamon, add eggs, milk, warmed butter, vanilla extract, and whip everything into a smooth dough. We can use a stick mixer. Pour the dough into a warm waffle maker and bake until pink. Meanwhile, whip the cottage cheese with cocoa and season with a spoonful protein drink hazelnut and chocolate. Finished waffles are served with whipped chocolate curd.

5. Cheese Keto Patties

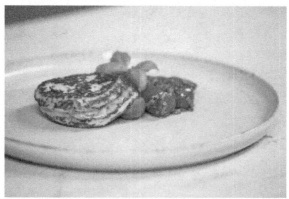

Servings: 2
Preparation time: 30 minutes
Ingredients

- Basil according to taste
- Herbs according to taste
- Cheddar - 2 slices
- Cherry tomatoes - 5 pcs

- KetoDiet protein omelet with cheese flavor - 1 bag
- Cauliflower - 300 g
- Olive oil according to taste
- Parmesan - 50 g
- Salt according to taste

Instructions
Salt the grated cauliflower, let it stand and drain the excess water and squeeze through a cloth. Thoroughly mix one serving of KetoDiet protein omelet (in a shaker or whisk) in 100 ml of water, mix with cauliflower, herbs, and grated Parmesan cheese. From the dough, we make patties, which we fry in a pan until browned; we put a cheddar slice and let it melt. We serve vegetable salads with pancakes, for example from cherry tomatoes with basil dripped with olive oil.

6. Keto Porridge with Wild Berries

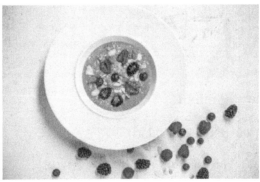

Servings: 1
Preparation time: 15 minutes
Ingredients
- chicory syrup according to taste
- KetoDiet raspberry porridge - 1 piece
- Coconut milk - 50 ml
- Forest fruit - 100 g
- Milk - 100 ml
- Almond slices - 1 tbsp
- Shredded coconut - 1 tbsp

- Cottage cheese ~ 1 tbsp

Instructions
Whip the protein raspberry porridge with the milk (cow and coconut) until smooth and put it in the microwave for a minute, or heat the milk in a saucepan and pour the contents of the bag into the hot milk and mix thoroughly. Stir 50 g of mixed forest fruit into the finished porridge, add coconut, a spoonful of cottage cheese and garnish with dry roasted almond slices and the remaining fruit.

7. Keto Potato Pancakes

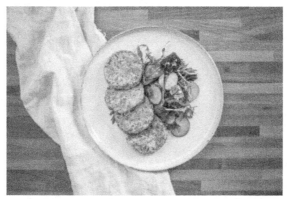

Servings: 1
Preparation time: 20 minutes
Ingredients

- Balsamic ~ 1 teaspoon (for salad)
- Celery ~ 150 g
- Garlic ~ 1 clove
- Crushed cumin according to taste
- KetoDiet protein pancake with garlic flavor ~ 1 serving
- Marjoram according to taste
- Ground flax seeds ~ 1 tablespoon
- Oil according to taste
- Olive oil ~ 1 tablespoon (for salad)
- Pepper according to taste
- Radish ~ 3 pcs (for salad)

- A mixture of green salads (arugula, romaine lettuce, corn salad) 1 handful (for salad)
- Salt according to taste
- Water - 100 ml

Instructions

Grate the celery and mix it with all the ingredients, including the protein pancake powder, to make a thinner dough. We make patties from the dough, which we fry until golden in a pan. Serve with a vegetable salad of mixed salad (we used corn on the cob, arugula, beet leaves), chopped radishes, which we cut. Mix everything and drizzle with the prepared dressing of olive oil and balsamic.

8. Baked Avocado

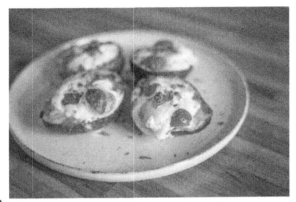

Servings: 2
Preparation time: 30 minutes
Ingredients

- Avocado - 2
- Cherry tomatoes to taste
- Pepper to taste
- Bacon - 4 slices
- Salt to taste
- Cottage cheese - 1
- Egg - 4 pieces

Instructions

Cut the avocado lengthwise and remove the stone. We dig out a little pulp with a spoon. Put the hollowed-out avocados in a small baking dish with baking paper. Tap 1 small egg in each half of the avocado and add a piece of bacon, cottage cheese, cherry tomatoes, etc. Add salt and pepper. Bake until the egg is ready.

9. Pasta Salad

Servings: 1
Preparation time: 20 minutes
Ingredients

- KetoDiet protein pasta Fusilli- 1 serving
- Olive oil - 2 tablespoons (for mayonnaise)
- Pepper according to taste
- Radish - 3 pcs
- Cucumber - 100 g
- A mixture of green salads (arugula, romaine lettuce, corn salad) 1 handful
- Salt according to taste
- Sour cream - 1 tablespoon (for mayonnaise)
- Green pepper - 100 g

Instructions
Cut peppers, cucumber, and radish and mix them with salad and ready-made protein pasta, which we cooked according to the instructions. Pour the homemade mayonnaise over the salad, which we prepare from sour cream, olive oil, salt, and pepper. Garnish with chives or herbs and serve.
ATTENTION! If you have this mayonnaise in step 1 of your diet plan, omit half the amount (= 1 DCL) of milk allowed that day.

10. Baked Keto Peppers

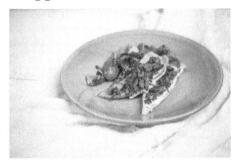

Servings: 2
Preparation time: 60 minutes
Ingredients

- Balsamic - 1 teaspoon (for salad)
- White or green pepper - 2 pcs
- Garlic - 1 clove
- Cherry tomatoes - 5 pcs (for salad)
- Half onion
- KetoDiet protein omelet with cheese flavor - 1 piece
- Ground beef meat - 100 g
- Olive oil - 20 ml for peppers + to taste for salad
- Pepper according to taste
- Radish - 5 pcs (for salad)
- Rosemary according to taste
- A mixture of green salads (arugula, romaine lettuce, corn salad), a handful (for salad)
- Salt according to taste
- Water - 100 ml
- Mushrooms - 3 pcs

Instructions
We clean the pepper, cut it in half, and get rid of the kernels. Fry the sliced mushrooms with a sprig of rosemary in a hot pan and set them aside. Now fry the chopped onion in the same pan, add the minced meat, garlic and season with salt and pepper. Once the meat is roasted, add the mushrooms to the mixture and mix.

Fill the halved peppers with the meat mixture and pour them over the water with a mixed protein omelet—Bake in a baking dish at 150 ° C for about 20 minutes. Serve with a vegetable salad of 5 cherry tomatoes, 5 radishes, and a handful of mixed salad, which we drizzle with a dressing of 1 tablespoon olive oil, 1 teaspoon balsamic, salt and pepper.

11. Easter Lamb

Servings: 6
Preparation time: 0 minutes
Ingredients

- Chicory syrup - 1/4 cup
- 1/2 lemon juice
- KetoDiet Protein Drink - 1 serving
- Baking powder - 1 piece
- Almond flour - 1 and 1/4 cup
- Ground flax seeds - 1/2 cup
- Ground poppy seeds - 1/2 cup
- Greek white yogurt - 1 mug
- Egg - 4 pieces

Instructions
Mix Greek yogurt, add almond flour, 1 serving of protein drink, eggs, mixed flax seeds, poppy seeds, lemon juice, chicory syrup, and 1 baking powder. Mix everything well and pour into the erased form—Bake for about 40 minutes at 180 ° C.

12. Keto Tart with Wild Berries

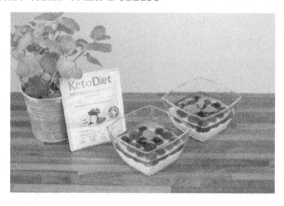

Servings: 2
Preparation: 60 minutes
Ingredients

- Chicory syrup - 1 tablespoon
- KetoDiet protein panna cotta - 1 serving
- Forest fruit - 200 g
- Mascarpone - 100 g
- Mint for decoration
- Whole cottage cheese - 100 g
- Gelatin - 1 piece

Instructions

Mix mascarpone with cottage cheese and protein panna cotta mixture and sweeten with chicory syrup. Pour the finished cream into a bowl and place the forest fruits on top. Pour the prepared gelatin according to the instructions and let it cool in the refrigerator until the gelatin hardens. Decorate with a sprig of mint, for example.

Lunch

1. Keto Pasta Curry

Servings: 2
Preparation time: 30 minutes
Ingredients

- Fresh baby spinach a handful of petals
- Fresh coriander according to taste
- Garlic - 1 clove
- Zucchini - 100 g
- Curry spice according to taste
- KetoDiet protein cheese soup with vegetables - 1 bag
- KetoDiet protein pasta Fusilli - 1 bag
- Coconut milk - 50 ml
- Oil according to taste
- Shallot - 1
- Water - 170 ml

Instructions

Fry finely chopped onion, crushed garlic, chopped zucchini, and curry in oil and sauté until soft. Mix KetoDiet protein cheese soup in hot water, add to the mixture and cook for a while. Mix with Fusilli protein pasta cooked according to the instructions, spinach, pour coconut milk and sprinkle with coriander.

2. Vegetable-Mushroom Keto Omelette

Serving: 1
Preparation time: 20 minutes
Ingredients

- Fresh baby spinach, a handful of petals
- Zucchini ~100 g
- Pumpkin ~ 100 g
- KetoDiet Protein omelet with bacon flavor ~ 1 serving
- Oil according to taste
- Parmesanfor sprinkling
- Pepper according to taste
- Salt according to taste
- Mushrooms ~ 50 g

Instructions

Cut zucchini, pumpkin, and mushrooms into pieces, fry in oil, salt, pepper, add spinach leaves. Mix the KetoDiet protein omelet in water, pour over the vegetables, sprinkle with cheese, and bake for 5~10 minutes at 180 ° C.

3. Avocado Foam

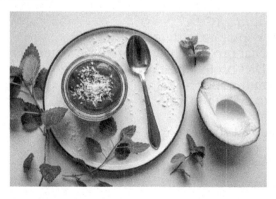

Serving: 1
Preparation time: 15 min
Ingredients

- Avocado - 1/2
- Cocoa - 2 tablespoons
- Coconut milk - 20 ml
- KetoDiet protein drink flavored with hazelnut and chocolate - 10 g
- Shredded coconut - 1 tbsp

Instructions
Dissolve one tablespoon (10 g) of flavored protein drink (vanilla or hazelnut flavor and chocolate) in coconut milk, add skinless and stone-free avocado, cocoa and mix into a smooth cream. Serve sprinkled with grated coconut.

4. Keto Specle with Spinach

Servings: 2
Preparation: 30 minutes
Ingredients

- Fresh baby spinach handful
- Garlic - 1 clove
- KetoDiet protein omelet with cheese flavor - 1 bag
- Baking powder - 1/2 teaspoon
- Olive oil according to taste
- Parmesan - 25 g
- Shallot - 1/2
- Whipping cream - 50 ml
- Salt according to taste
- Cottage cheese - 1 tbsp
- Egg - 1

Instructions
Beat eggs with cottage cheese, baking powder, and powder from a bag with KetoDiet omelet. Pour the resulting dough into a decorating bag and make speckles into boiling salted water—Cook for about 3 minutes. Pour the cooked specks and fry dry until golden in a hot pan.

Place the finished speckles on a plate and fry the finely chopped onion, garlic in the pan and fry for a while. Return the speckle to the pan, mix, pour over the cream, mix in the baby spinach and finally sprinkle with grated Parmesan cheese.

5. Keto Mushrooms with Celery Fries

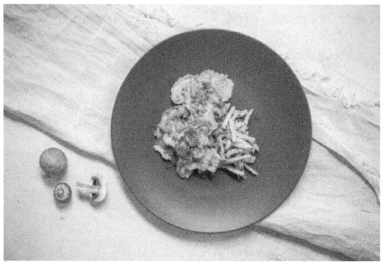

Servings: 1
Preparation: 40 minutes
Ingredients

- Herbs for decoration
- Celery ~ 200 g
- KetoDiet Protein omelet with bacon flavor ~ 1 serving
- Olive oil ~ 2 tbsp
- Pepper according to taste
- Salt according to taste
- Water ~ 100 ml
- Mushrooms ~ 3 pcs

Instructions
Clean the celery, cut it into thin fries, drizzle with olive oil, salt, pepper, and bake in the oven for about 15 minutes at 165 ° C. We watch the french fries in the oven because it depends on how strong we cut them.

Meanwhile, cut the mushrooms into slices and mix them with the protein omelet mixed in water. The mushrooms wrapped "in batter" from an omelet are then sautéed until golden in oil. We can pour the rest of the omelet on the mushroom pan so that we don't miss a bit of protein. Serve with celery fries.

6. Turkey Roll with Spring Onion, Olives, and Sun-Dried tomatoes

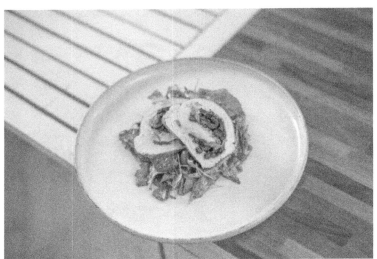

Servings: 4
Preparation time: 80 minutes
Ingredients

- Balsamic to taste
- Black olives - 60 g
- Garlic - 20 g
- Cherry tomatoes - 280 g
- Spring onion - 120 g
- Turkey breast - 400 g
- Olive oil - 40 ml
- Pepper to taste
- Rocket - 120 g
- Salt to taste
- Dried tomatoes in oil - 60 g

Instructions

Carefully cut the turkey breast lengthwise so that a larger pancake is formed and tap the meat. Fry the finely chopped spring onion and garlic in a pan in olive oil. Add olives cut in half and sliced sun-dried tomatoes, and fry everything briefly.

Apply the mixture to a slice of turkey meat and carefully roll it into a roll. Tie with thread and bake at 180 degrees for 50 minutes. Cut the finished roll into slices and serve with arugula salad and fresh cherry tomatoes flavored with olive oil and balsamic.

7. Zucchini Lasagna

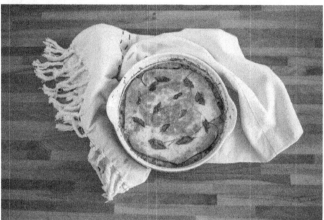

Servings: 2
Preparation time: 60 minutes
Ingredients
- Basil as required
- Red wine - 1 glass
- Onion - 1
- Zucchini - 1
- Ground beef - 250 g
- Olive oil as required
- Pepper to taste
- Tomatoes - 1 can (without added sugar)
- Whipping cream - 1 piece
- Grated cheddar to taste
- Salt to taste
- Egg - 1 piece

Instructions

Fry the diced onion in olive oil, add the minced meat, salt, pepper, add basil and sauté.

Once the meat has pulled, cover with red wine and stew. When the wine boils, add chopped tomatoes, cover, and simmer for about 30 minutes. Cut the zucchini lengthwise into thin slices. It works best with a potato peeler, but we can also playfully handle it with a knife. Wipe the baking dish with butter, layout the zucchini slices, pour the sauce over the minced meat, sprinkle with grated cheddar, and pour over the beaten egg in the cream. Layer another layer of zucchini, sauce, cheddar, and pour again with cream and egg. We repeat the whole thing, and we finish with a layer of cheddar and cream. Bake in a preheated oven at 200 degrees for about 30 minutes.

8. Keto Soup with Zucchini

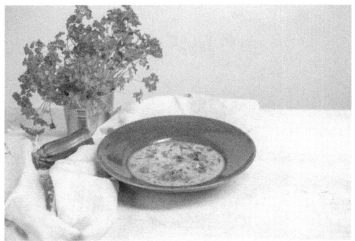

Servings: 1
Preparations: 15 minutes
Ingredients

- Herbs according to taste
- Garlic - 1 clove
- Onion - 1/2 pcs
- Zucchini - 150 g
- KetoDiet protein cheese soup with vegetables - 1 piece
- Butter - 1 teaspoon
- Olive oil - 20 ml
- Pepper according to taste
- Water - 250 ml

Instructions

In a small saucepan, fry the zucchini chopped in olive oil, add salt, pepper, herbs, and garlic. Pour water and cook until soft. Finally, stir in the cheese protein soup, a teaspoon of butter, turn off the flame and let it run for 3 minutes. Garnish with herbs.

9. Pumpkin with Greek Feta Cheese

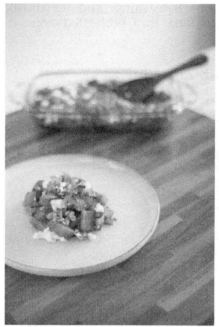

Servings: 2
Preparation time: 85 minutes
Ingredients

- Hokaido pumpkins - 1
- Olive oil as required
- Pepper to taste
- Sunflower seeds to taste
- Garlic cloves - 3
- Salt to taste
- Feta cheese - 100 g
- Thyme - 2 sprigs
- Walnuts as required

Instructions

Peel the pumpkin, remove the seeds, cut into larger cubes, and spread in a baking dish. We don't peel garlic, so let's avoid burning it. Bake the mixture for about 40 minutes at 180 degrees, then add the walnuts and sunflower seeds and bake gently for about 10 minutes. We do not add nuts sooner so that they do not burn. Take the baked goods out of the oven and sprinkle with grated feta cheese. To make the cheese beautifully baked, put it in the oven for another 5 minutes.

10. Keto Houstičky with Herb Butter

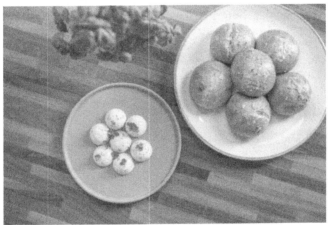

Serving: 3
Preparation time: 60 minutes
Ingredients

- White - 3 pcs
- Herbs to taste (for herb butter)
- Pumpkin seeds - 1 tbsp
- Hot water - 1/2 cup
- Apple vinegar - 2 teaspoons
- KetoDiet Protein Drink - 2 servings
- Baking powder - 2 teaspoons
- Gourmet yeast - 2 tablespoons
- Almond flour - 1 and 1/4 cup
- Butter - 4 tablespoons (for herb butter)
- Psyllium (fiber) - 5 tablespoons

- Sunflower or flax seeds - 1 tbsp
- Salt - 1 teaspoon
- Maldon saltfor sprinkling
- Yolk - 1 piece

Instructions

Mix the ingredients, including the protein powder, and add hot water while whipping constantly. Add a pinch of salt, stir again. We shape 6 buns from the dough and place on a baking sheet. We leave gaps between them, because the pastry will increase in volume during baking. Brush the buns with egg yolk and bake for about 30 minutes at 160 ° C. Let the finished buns cool down and serve them with herb butter, for example, which we prepare by mixing herbs according to your taste into the softened butter and letting them harden to any shape in the fridge. We used parsley, basil, and thyme.

11. Baked Keto Fennel

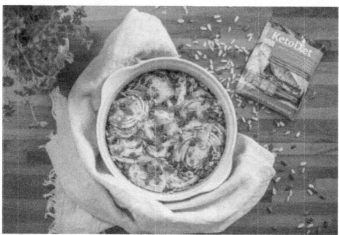

Servings: 2
Preparation time: 70 minutes
Ingredients
- Fresh fennel - 2 bulbs
- Pumpkin seeds - 2 tablespoons
- KetoDiet protein omelet with cheese flavor - 1 serving
- Olive oil - 1 tablespoon
- Chive according to taste
- Pepper according to taste

- Parsley according to taste
- Sunflower seeds - 2 tablespoons
- Whipping cream - 150 ml
- Salt according to taste
- Hard cheese - 50 g

Instructions
Wash and cut the fennel into slices, which we place in a baking dish. Season with salt, pepper, herbs, and mix with olive oil. Pour in a protein omelet mixed in cream, cover with grated cheese and bake at 165 ° C for about 50 minutes. Meanwhile, fry the pumpkin and sunflower seeds dry in a pan and sprinkle them on the finished meal. Garnish with, for example, the remaining herbs or sprigs of fennel.

12. Wholemeal Couscous with Cherry Tomatoes

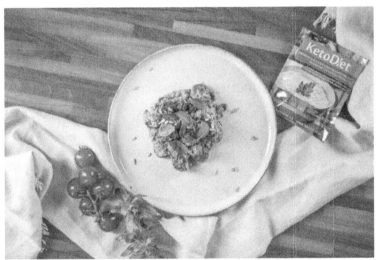

Serving: 1
Preparation time: 20 minutes
Ingredients
- Wholegrain couscous - 50 g
- Fresh basil handful
- Garlic - 1 clove
- Cherry tomatoes - 5 pcs
- Half Zucchini
- KetoDiet chicken/beef protein soup (depends on your taste) 1 bag

- Olive oil - 1 tbsp
- Parmesan - 30 g
- Sunflower seeds - 2 spoons for pesto + 1 spoon for decoration
- Water - 100 ml

Instructions

Prepare the protein soup in 100 ml of water and let it stand for 3 minutes. Pour the finished soup over the dry couscous and let stand for another 5 minutes to soak up the couscous. Meanwhile, cut the zucchini into rounds, fry it dry on both sides in a pan, add olive oil, tomatoes, and garlic and fry the mixture. Add the finished couscous, a spoonful of pesto, and mix. Garnish with fresh basil, a little pesto, and roasted sunflower seeds and serve. How to make homemade basil pesto? Very simple! We mix a handful of basil, 2 tablespoons of sunflower seeds, 2 tablespoons of olive oil, and 2 tablespoons of grated Parmesan cheese and decorate the finished couscous with it.

Dinner

1. Keto Pasta with Zucchini

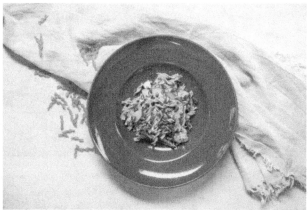

Servings: 1
Preparation time: 20 minutes
Ingredients

- Fresh parsley according to taste
- Garlic - 1 clove
- Zucchini - 120 g

- Pumpkin seeds - 1 tbsp
- KetoDiet protein pasta Fusilli - 1 piece
- Olive oil - 1 tbsp
- Salt according to taste
- The egg white - 1 piece

Instructions

Cut the zucchini into pieces. Fry the pumpkin seeds dry in a pan. Pour the seeds into a bowl and fry finely chopped or pressed garlic in oil and add the zucchini. Once the zucchini softens, add the cooked protein pasta according to the instructions and pour over the protein. Salt and mix until the pasta is slightly combined with the zucchini and the egg whites. Finally, sprinkle with fried pumpkin seeds and garnish with parsley.

2. Keto Pizza

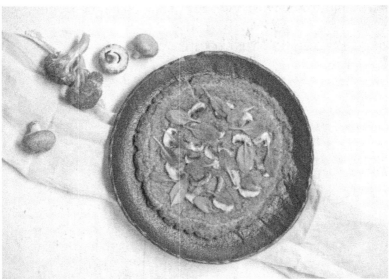

Servings: 1 serving
Preparation time: 60 minutes
Ingredients

- Broccoli - 250 g
- Fresh baby spinach handful (for lining)
- Garlic - 1 clove (for lining)
- KetoDiet Protein Drink - 1 scoop (15 g)

- Oregano to taste (for dough and lining)
- Parmesan - 10 g
- Parmesan for sprinkling
- Pepper according to taste
- Tomatoes - 2 pcs (for lining)
- Egg - 1 piece
- Mushrooms - 2 pcs (for lining)

Instructions

We break down the broccoli into roses, which we mix in a small mixer. Spread the broccoli on a baking sheet lined and bake for 10 minutes in an oven preheated to 180 ° C. Mix baked broccoli with egg, protein drink, and grated parmesan, salt, and pepper. Make a pancake from the dough, spread a mixture of mixed tomatoes, garlic, and oregano on it. Put with sliced mushrooms and lightly sprinkle with grated Parmesan cheese. Bake the pizza at 180 ° C for about 15 minutes. Garnish with baby spinach before serving.

3. Baked Portobello Mushrooms

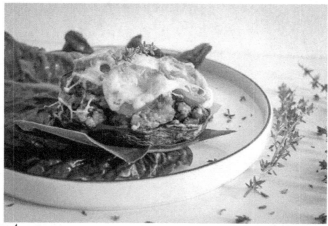

Servings: 4
Preparation time: 30 minutes
Ingredients

- Red onion - 1
- Garlic according to taste
- Cherry tomatoes - 4

- Goat cheese - 150 g
- Ground beef - 250 g
- Pepper according to taste
- Vegetable oil according to need
- Salt according to taste
- Thyme according to taste
- Portobello mushroom - 4

Instructions

We clean the heads of mushrooms, remove the foot and hollow out the inside, cut the foot into smaller pieces. Heat oil in a pan and add minced meat, thyme, crushed garlic, salt, pepper, and sauté for a while. Add the inside of the mushroom and a sliced leg to the meat. Fill the finished mixture with mushroom caps, place the sliced red onion, sliced cherry tomatoes on the wheels, and sprinkle with grated cheese. Bake for 25 minutes in an oven heated to 180 ° C. Mushrooms are served with fresh vegetable salad.

4. Baked Protein Omelette

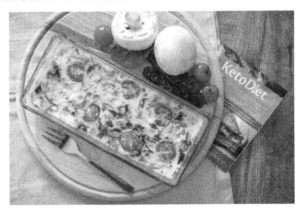

Serving: 1
Preparation time: 30 minutes
Ingredients

- Cherry tomatoes - 2
- Zucchini - 50 g
- KetoDiet cheese omelette - 1
- Chard - 20 g
- Pepper according to taste

- Vegetable oil according to need
- Salt according to taste
- Hard cheese (up to 30% fat in dry matter) - 50 g
- Mushrooms - 50 g

Instructions

Cut the zucchini into pieces, slice the mushrooms, salt, pepper and fry together for a while in hot oil; add the sliced chard leaf, mix and put in a baking dish. In the shaker, mix the protein omelet according to the instructions and pour on the mixture. Add chopped cherry tomatoes and sprinkle with grated cheese—Bake for about 25 minutes at 180 ° C.

5. Zucchini Pie

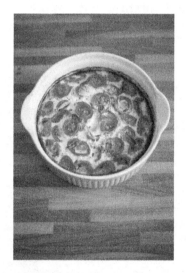

Servings: 4
Preparation time: 60 minutes
Ingredients

- Basil to taste
- Zucchini - 1
- Mozzarella - 1
- Pepper to taste
- Salt to taste
- Egg - 3

Instructions

In a bowl, mix 1 larger mozzarella with 3 eggs. Grate the zucchini, mix everything, salt, and pepper. Pour into a baking dish. Garnish the slices of tomato on top, we can also add fresh basil leaves. Bake at a temperature of 180 degrees for about 30-40 minutes.

6. Salad with Olives and Cottage Cheese

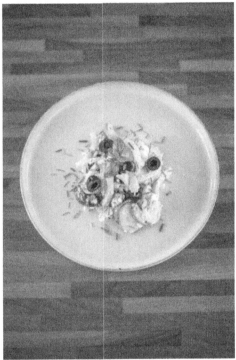

Serving: 1
Preparation time: 15 minutes
Ingredients

- Black olives as required
- Cucumber salad - 1/2
- Pepper - 1
- Pepper to taste
- Tomatoes - 2
- Salt to taste
- Cottage cheese - 1

Instructions

Cut the vegetables into cubes, add the black olives to taste, salt, pepper, and mix with 1 cup of cottage cheese. Sprinkle with finely chopped chives on top.

7. Vegetable Salad with Goat Cheese

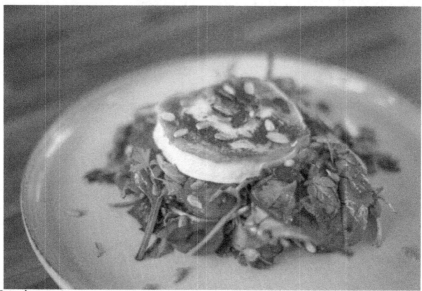

Servings: 2
Preparation time: 30 minutes
Ingredients
- Balsamic - 1 tablespoon
- Cherry tomatoes as required
- Goat cheese - 2 slices
- Olive oil - 2 tablespoons + for dripping
- Seed mixture (sunflower, pumpkin) - 1 package
- A mixture of green salads (arugula, romaine lettuce, corn salad) - 1 package

Instructions

Cut goat cheese into thicker slices and grill or fry dry in a non-stick pan. Mix popular types of green salads with cherry tomatoes and season with a mixture of olive oil and balsamic. We can taste it with a pinch of salt and, depending on the taste, also pepper. Place the roasted goat cheese slices on a salad, sprinkle with a mixture of seeds and drizzle with olive oil.

Desserts

1. Keto Panna Cotta with Wild Berries

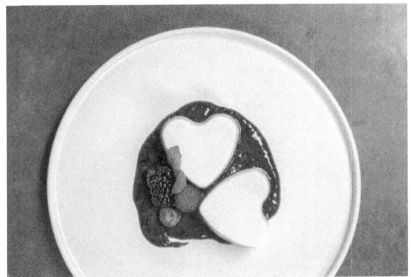

Servings: 1
Preparation time: 80 minutes
Ingredients
- Forest fruit - 100 g
- Milk - 100 ml
- Protein panna cotta with cream and vanilla flavor - 1 bag

Instructions
According to the instructions, mix the protein panna cotta in milk, pour it into a mold, and let it solidify in the refrigerator. Pour the finished panna cotta onto a plate and garnish with mixed forest fruits and a sprig of mint.

2. Sweet Potato-Pumpkin Christmas Salad

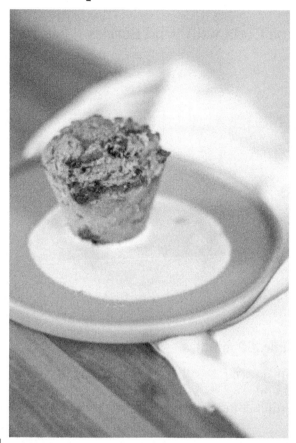

Servings: 4
Preparation time: 60 minutes
Ingredients
- Sweet potatoes - 2 pieces
- Chili spice pinch if you like spicy dishes
- Spring onion one volume
- Gherkin, according to taste
- A smaller butter pumpkin or a smaller Hokaido pumpkin 1 piece
- Pepper according to taste
- Whole mustard - 3 tbsp
- Salt according to taste
- Egg - 4 pieces

Instructions

Cut the pumpkin, carve it out and cut into the same smaller cubes. We also peel and dice sweet potatoes into cubes (we select larger pieces). We cook everything in salted water for about 10 minutes. Drain the water and let it cool completely. Meanwhile, we boil the eggs hard, peel them, and cut them into cubes. We also finely chop pickles and spring onions. We definitely do not miss it; it will give the salad a great taste. Mix everything, salt, pepper, season with mustard, and mayonnaise. The salad will be better if we let it cool down and rest a little.

3. Unbaked Cheesecake in a glass

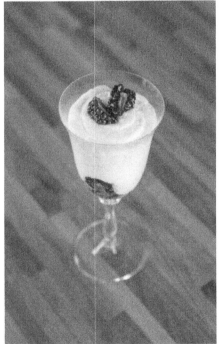

Servings: 8
Preparation time: 20 minutes
Ingredients

- chicory syrup to taste
- Mascarpone - 1
- Blackberries for decoration
- Whipped cream - 1 (whipped)
- Philadelphia cheese - 1 package

Instructions

Carefully mix the cheese and whipped cream with chicory syrup and pour into the prepared glasses. Garnish with blueberries or strawberries. Let cool in the fridge for at least an hour.

4. Chocolate Muesli Balls with Nuts

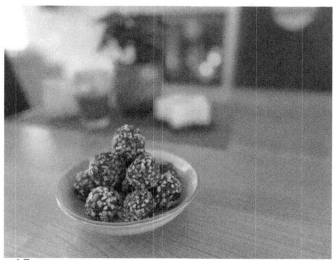

Servings: 15
Preparation: 30 minutes
Ingredients
- 70% dark chocolate - 25 g
- Fine muesli KetoLife - 150 g
- Hazelnuts - 30 g
- Butter - 70 g
- Protein cream with hazelnuts - 100 g

Instructions

From fine muesli, protein cream with hazelnuts (we use either 2 smaller packages of cream or 5 tablespoons from a large package), and melted butter, we create a dough from which we form balls. Put 1 hazelnut in each and wrap in melted 70% chocolate and chopped hazelnuts. We store the balls in the refrigerator.

5. Sweet Potato Muffins

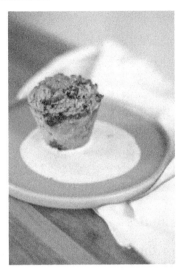

Servings: 3
Preparation time: 50 minutes
Ingredients
- Sweet potatoes - 250 g
- Blueberries handful
- Chicory syrup to taste
- KetoDiet protein mixture - 2 measuring cups
- Baking powder - 1 bag
- Almond flour - 25 g
- Cinnamon - 1 tbsp
- Egg - 4
- Walnuts - 2 tablespoons (ground)

Instructions
Thoroughly mix the grated muffins with other ingredients, or mix and pour into molds (6 pcs). Bake at 180 degrees for 15-20 minutes until golden brown.

6. Walnut-Chocolate Balls

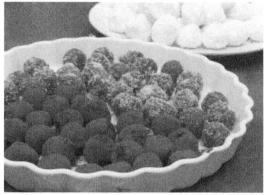

Servings: 12
Preparation time: 30 minutes
Ingredients
- Chicory syrup according to taste
- Hot chocolate - 100 g
- Cocoa for wrapping
- Coconut for wrapping
- Butter according to need
- Rum aroma according to taste
- Cinnamon for wrapping
- Walnuts - 250 g

Instructions
For 50 balls. Grind the nuts, mix with melted chocolate, butter, rum aroma, syrup. We make balls from the dough, which we wrap in cinnamon, cocoa, or coconut.

7. Chocolate Laundries

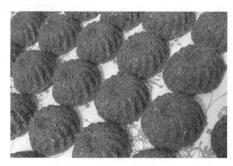

Servings: 5

Preparation time: 45 minutes
Ingredients
- Birch sugar xylitol - 3 tablespoons
- Cocoa - 3 tablespoons
- Baking powder - 1 teaspoon
- Almond flour - 70 g
- Butter - 35 g
- Dried whey - 20 g
- Egg yolk - 2

Instructions
We mix all the ingredients and work out the dough with our hands, which we press into the laundries' molds—Bake in the oven at 180 ° C for about 8 minutes.

8. Coconuts in Chocolate

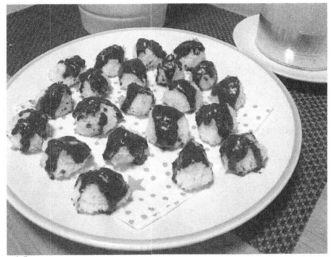

Servings: 12
Preparation time: 45 minutes
Ingredients

- Hot chocolate according to need

- Whole cottage cheese8 tablespoons

- Shredded coconut - 200 g

- The egg white - 4

Instructions

We whip the snow from the proteins. Mix the ingredients in a bowl and use a spoon to form balls, which we bake on baking paper at a temperature of 160 ° C until golden. Soak in melted chocolate.

9. Linen Wheels

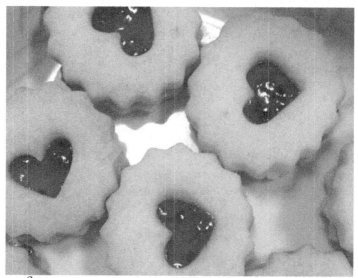

Servings: 6
Preparation time: 45 minutes
Ingredients
- Chicory syrup - 3 tablespoons
- Baking powder - 1 teaspoon
- Almond flour - 70 g
- Butter - 35 g
- Dried whey - 20 g
- Egg yolk - 2 pcs

Instructions
From these ingredients, we make a dough, which we leave to rest in the fridge for several hours. Then roll out on a thin pancake and cut out the wheels or hearts as you wish. Bake on baking paper at 170 ° C for about 10 minutes. After cooling, combine with jam or chocolate cream without sugar.

10. Almond Balls

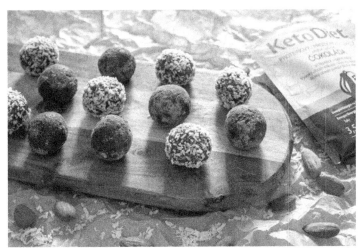

Servings: 4
Preparation time: 50 minutes
Ingredients

- Cocoa - 2 tablespoons
- KetoDiet Protein Drink - 2 tablespoons
- Almond flour - 3 tablespoons
- Almond butter - 3 tablespoons
- Shredded coconut - 2 tablespoons

Instructions
Mix almond butter, ground nuts, grated coconut, cocoa powder, and a chocolate-flavored protein drink and work everything into the dough. Divide into 12 equal parts, from which we form balls. We then wrap the individual balls in coconut and cocoa powder.

CHAPTER 5

30-Day Meal Plan

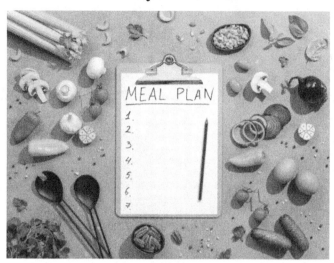

Week 1

Day One
Breakfast: Chorizo Breakfast Bake
Lunch: Sesame Pork Lettuce Wraps
Dinner: Avocado Lime Salmon

Day Two
Breakfast: Keto Potato Pancakes
Lunch: Keto Pasta Curry
Dinner: Leftover Avocado Lime Salmon

Day Three
Breakfast: Baked Eggs in Avocado
Lunch: Easy Beef Curry
Dinner: Veggies and Rosemary Roasted Chicken

Day Four
Breakfast: Lemon Poppy Ricotta Pancakes with 3 Slices Thick-Cut Bacon
Lunch: Zucchini lasagna

Dinner: Leftover Rosemary Roasted Chicken and Veggies

Day Five
Breakfast: Leftover Lemon Poppy Ricotta Pancakes with 3 Slices Thick-Cut Bacon
Lunch: Keto Pasta Curry
Dinner: Cheesy Sausage Mushroom Skillet with 1 Slice Thick-Cut Bacon

Day Six
Breakfast: Sweet Blueberry Coconut Porridge with 1 Slice Thick-Cut Bacon
Lunch: Avocado foam
Dinner: Baked portobello mushrooms

Day Seven
Breakfast: Leftover Sweet Blueberry Coconut Porridge
Lunch: Keto soup with zucchini
Dinner: Keto Pasta with Zucchini

Week 2

Day One
Breakfast: Banana Keto Chia Pudding
Lunch: Easy Cheeseburger Salad
Dinner: Chicken Zoodle Alfredo

Day Two
Breakfast: Savory Ham and Cheese Waffles with 2 Slices Thick-Cut Bacon
Lunch: Keto Pasta Curry
Dinner: Cabbage and Sausage Skillet

Day Three
Breakfast: Keto Potato Pancakes
Lunch: Pumpkin with Greek feta cheese
Dinner: Baked portobello mushrooms

Day Four
Breakfast: Keto Waffles with Chocolate Cottage Cheese
Lunch: Avocado foam
Dinner: Zucchini pie

Day Five
Breakfast: Keto Potato Pancakes
Lunch: Sausage Skillet and Cabbage
Dinner: Keto Pasta with Zucchini

Day Six
Breakfast: Matcha Keto Pudding
Lunch: Vegetable-mushroom Keto Omelette
Dinner: Zucchini pie

Day Seven
Breakfast: Keto Tart with wild berries
Lunch: Pumpkin with Greek feta cheese
Dinner: Salad with olives and Cottage cheese

Week 3

Day One
Breakfast: Green Keto Smoothie
Lunch: Mozzarella Tuna Melt
Dinner: Cheesy Single-Serve Lasagna

Day Two
Breakfast: Bacon Breakfast Bombs
Lunch: Avocado, Salami Sandwiches, and Egg
Dinner: Crispy Chipotle Chicken Thighs

Day Three
Breakfast: Keto Waffles with Chocolate Cottage Cheese
Lunch: Keto Pasta Curry
Dinner: Ham, Pepperoni, and Cheese Stromboli

Day Four
Breakfast: Matcha Keto Pudding
Lunch: Avocado foam
Dinner: Cheese Stromboli, Leftover Pepperoni and Ham

Day Five
Breakfast: Keto Tart with wild berries
Lunch: Keto Pasta Curry
Dinner: Keto Pasta with Zucchini

Day Six
Breakfast: Three-Cheese Pizza Frittata with 2 Slices Thick-Cut Bacon
Lunch: Keto Pasta Curry
Dinner: Spring Salad with Steak and Sweet Dressing

Day Seven
Breakfast: Leftover Three-Cheese Pizza Frittata with 2 Slices Thick-Cut Bacon
Lunch: Vegetable-mushroom Keto Omelette
Dinner: Keto Pasta with Zucchini

Week 4

Day One
Breakfast: Keto Tart with wild berries
Lunch: Zucchini Pasta Salad and Chicken
Dinner: *Carb Up* Flank Steak, Watermelon Salad, and Plantains
Snacks: Mojito Water

Day Two
Breakfast: Keto Tart with wild berries
Lunch: Keto Mushrooms with celery fries
Dinner: Chicken and Bacon with Slaw
Snacks: Tropical Coconut Balls

Day Three
Breakfast: Baked Keto Peppers
Lunch: Sardine Salad
Dinner: Chorizo Bowl
Snacks: Jicama Fries

Day Four
Breakfast: Rocket Fuel Latte with Maca
Lunch: Zucchini Pasta Salad and Chicken
Dinner: Keto Pasta with Zucchini
Snacks: Mojito Water

Day Five
Breakfast: Pasta Salad
Lunch: Vanilla Creme Gummies
Dinner: Salad with olives and Cottage cheese
Snacks: Jicama Fries

Day Six
Breakfast: Veggie Frittata
Lunch: Sardine Salad
Dinner: Chicken and Bacon with Slaw
Snacks: Tropical Coconut Balls

Day Seven
Breakfast: Baked Keto Peppers
Lunch: Chicken and Zucchini Pasta Salad
Dinner: Keto Pasta with Zucchini
Snacks: Mojito Water

Week 5

Day One
Breakfast: Mozzarella Veggie-Loaded Quiche with 1 Slice Thick-Cut Bacon
Lunch: Keto Pasta Curry
Dinner: Salad with olives and Cottage cheese

Day Two
Breakfast: Keto Tart with wild berries
Lunch: Vegetable-mushroom Keto Omelette
Dinner: Keto Pasta with Zucchini

CONCLUSION

The ketogenic diet can offer benefits to women during menopause, including increased sensitivity to insulin, decreased weight gain, and decreased cravings.

It can, however, increase some cardiovascular disease risk factors and reduce the intake of many essential nutrients. What's more, during your body's transition to ketosis, keto flu can temporarily exacerbate the symptoms of menopause.

While the ketogenic diet can work during menopause for some women, bear in mind that it is not a one-size-fits-all solution for everyone.

It's a wise idea to consider other less restrictive ways to improve your health and meet your fitness goals before trying out the keto diet.

Made in the USA
Las Vegas, NV
01 March 2023

68314622R10052